Male Infertility: An Integrative Manual of Western and Chinese Medicine

Authored by

Giovanna Franconi

Internal Medicine, Department of Systems Medicine,
Tor Vergata University of Rome, Rome,
Italy

Male Infertility: An Integrative Manual of Western and Chinese Medicine

Author: Giovanna Franconi

ISBN (Online): 978-1-68108-663-7

ISBN (Print): 978-1-68108-664-4

© 2018, Bentham eBooks imprint.

Published by Bentham Science Publishers – Sharjah, UAE. All Rights Reserved.

General:

1. Any dispute or claim arising out of or in connection with this License Agreement or the Work (including non-contractual disputes or claims) will be governed by and construed in accordance with the laws of the U.A.E. as applied in the Emirate of Dubai. Each party agrees that the courts of the Emirate of Dubai shall have exclusive jurisdiction to settle any dispute or claim arising out of or in connection with this License Agreement or the Work (including non-contractual disputes or claims).
2. Your rights under this License Agreement will automatically terminate without notice and without the need for a court order if at any point you breach any terms of this License Agreement. In no event will any delay or failure by Bentham Science Publishers in enforcing your compliance with this License Agreement constitute a waiver of any of its rights.
3. You acknowledge that you have read this License Agreement, and agree to be bound by its terms and conditions. To the extent that any other terms and conditions presented on any website of Bentham Science Publishers conflict with, or are inconsistent with, the terms and conditions set out in this License Agreement, you acknowledge that the terms and conditions set out in this License Agreement shall prevail.

Bentham Science Publishers Ltd.
Executive Suite Y - 2
PO Box 7917, Saif Zone
Sharjah, U.A.E.
Email: subscriptions@benthamscience.org

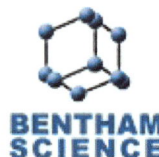

BENTHAM SCIENCE

CONTENTS

FOREWORD 1

As mankind has entered the 21st century, the natural ecological and social environment on Earth has undergone major changes, people's ideas of their own health have also been constantly updated, which makes modern medicine facing more challenges.

Andrology is a new science that studies the structure and function, physiology and pathology of male reproductive system. It is a branch of medical science that combines the basic and clinical research, and involves multidisciplinary mutual penetration. In recent years, great progress has been made in treatment of the male reproductive disorders and sexual dysfunction.

Male infertility is a complex problem, it can be only solved by bringing together medical wisdom and clinical experience of people all over the world.

He Jialang
Italian Institute of Traditional Chinese Medicine
Zhejiang Chinese Medical University
P.R. China

and

World Federation of Chinese Medicine Societies
Rome, Italy

FOREWORD 2

Infertility—for those who yearn for a child—may be the source of prolonged pain and suffering. Treatment which offers help to the infertile is therefore one of the highest forms of medicine.

Both in modern biomedicine and in traditional Chinese medicine, however, the focus has mostly been on the female partner. There is partial justification for this since a healthily fertile woman can compensate to some degree for impaired fertility in the male. Yet often the failure to address the male component of couple infertility reveals a deeper pattern of marginalising male health—a problem almost entirely created of course by men themselves. This failure is especially significant in a world where male fertility is declining in most animal species, including humans.

As we know from Chinese philosophy, we need to cultivate both yin and yang, and there is ample evidence that male infertility or subfertility is a factor in up to half of all couple infertility. And there are several benefits to be found in addressing the male partner. Firstly, underlying diseases and patterns of disharmony (as recognized in Chinese medicine) may be discovered and treated, benefiting a man's broader health and wellbeing. Secondly, successful treatment of male infertility may reduce the onus on the female to take fertility enhancing medication which may cause unwanted side effects. And finally, of course, the chances of a successful pregnancy will be increased if the male partner is treated as well as the female.

The treatment of female infertility has been the greatest success story in China's integration of cutting edge biomedicine with its long and rich medical traditions. This combined medicine now stands as probably the world's most successful and powerful approach to achieving successful pregnancies.

What has been missing, however, is an equivalent approach to treating male factor infertility, and practitioners have been unable to find a comprehensive and integrated account for both Western and Chinese medical approaches. Missing until now, that is, with the publication of Giovanna Franconi's welcome Male Infertility: An Integrative Manual of Western Medicine and Chinese Medicine.

This is the kind of book that should make the Western Chinese medicine profession proud, offering as it does a clear and comprehensive manual for the enhancement of fertility, which is the vital source of life.

Peter Deadman
Founder and Editor, Journal of Chinese Medicine
Author, Manual of Acupuncture
Author, Live Well Live Long
UK

PREFACE

Infertility is a problem that adversely affects the quality of life for a growing number of couples. Clinically defined as the inability of a sexually active couple to achieve pregnancy spontaneously within a year, it affects about one couple in every five. The advent of IntraCytoplasmic Sperm Injection (ICSI) has revolutionized infertility treatment, in particular for the male factor. Nevertheless, it continues to be important to properly assess infertile men to identify any infertility conditions that can be potentially corrected, in order to avoid the use of procedures of Assisted Reproduction Techniques (ART) whenever possible. On the other hand, even if some conditions of irreversible infertility can be treated with ART, it is important to identify those cases where this is not possible, saving the biological and psychological cost of ineffective therapies to the couple. The objective of the evaluation of the infertile male should also include, in addition to sperm recovery, the optimization of the reproductive potential in order to use less invasive reproductive techniques. It is also important to identify certain specific genetic causes of male infertility, which allows the couple to be informed about the possibility of transmitting genetic abnormalities to their offspring. Finally, we must not forget that the infertile man is not a healthy man. The altered spermatogenesis, on the basis of epidemiological data, is correlated with an increased risk of testicular cancer—the most common cancer in the age group between 15 and 44 years—the incidence of which is increasing in Caucasian populations.

In recent decades more emphasis has been placed on the role of the male factor in couple infertility, but it is still not adequate. Despite the fact that the male factor alone is responsible for infertility in 20% of couples, and that together with the female factor it contributes to infertility in another 30–40% of cases, it often happens that infertile couples are evaluated only by a gynecologist, who may have not received specialized training regarding the male factor challenges.

Male infertility is idiopathic in 50–70% of cases, and therefore subject to a mostly empirical therapy with limited effectiveness. This therapeutic gap could benefit from other medical approaches which deal with health and disease using different approaches. Traditional Chinese Medicine (TCM) is one of the few comprehensive traditional medical systems in use in the world, and with its age-old traditions and its sophisticated diagnostic and treatment system it can make a great contribution to human health. Over the course of thousands of years, TCM has developed a complex conceptual and methodological framework to both diagnose and also treat male infertility. The problems related to infertility appear in the oldest texts of Chinese medicine, and a growing number of scientific publications are evaluating its efficacy in the field of infertility. TCM considers health and disease from a holistic point of view, based on the concept that the body is able to self-regulate and adapt to the environment. For these reasons, in many ART centres around the world the gynecologist and the andrologist are complemented by an acupuncturist to maximize the fertility potential of couples, effectively creating an integrated approach to infertility.

The Western medical system at this time is a system based on evidence, applying therapies that have been found effective in randomized controlled studies, in which it is demonstrated that an intervention with a particular drug induces a greater therapeutic response than a placebo. The traditional Chinese medical system, however, is a system based on experience: the transfer of empirical knowledge from teacher to student over generations for centuries suggests the safety and efficacy of treatments handed down by tradition.

This book originates from the fact that the integration of Western medicine and Chinese medicine is asked for and sought after by infertile couples, and it has been written to help treat an infertile man by a specialist in acupuncture and/or in Chinese medicine, but who has no specific specializations in andrology. It is a manual that can serve as a guide in the clinical evaluation of the infertile man, both from the etiopathogenic point of view to understand the causes of his infertility, and from the diagnostic point of view to evaluate and interpret the biochemical and instrumental tests, and from the therapeutic point of view to develop a rational and integrated treatment. The numerous and detailed Appendices and the extensive Bibliography provide direct access to the most important technical information of Western medicine and Chinese medicine, providing an information platform for orientation and treatment of male infertility.

This is not a self-treatment book, and the treatments should be recommended only by specialists in Traditional Chinese Medicine. The Chinese herbal formulas mentioned in the text are indicative, and it is the task of the doctor of TCM to carefully evaluate indications, contraindications and incompatibility of individual herbs and formulas in each case. Also, local legislations which may have introduced restrictions on the use of various remedies of the Chinese pharmacopoeia should be checked.

Quotations from the Su Wen are from the book by Paul Unschuld [1], and those from Lingshu are taken from Van Nghi's book [2]. While the publisher and the author have used their best efforts in preparing this book, they make no representations or warranties with respect to the accuracy or completeness of the contents of this book and specifically disclaim any implied warranties of merchantability or fitness for a particular purpose. No warranty may be created or extended by sales representatives or written sales materials. The advice and strategies contained herein may not be suitable for your situation. You should consult with a professional where appropriate. Neither the publisher nor the author shall be liable for any loss of profit or any other commercial damages, including but not limited to special, incidental, consequential, or other damages.

This manual is based on the direct and indirect contribution of many, whom I thank here following a purely alphabetical order: Rosa Brotzu, Dante De Berardinis, Carlo Di Stanislao, Jlenia Elia, Andrea Fabbri, Giovanni Giambalvo Dal Ben, Mario Goncalves, Henry Johannes Greten, Paola Innocenzi, Csilla Krausz, Li Hong, Mario Maggi, Luigi Manni, Ferdinand Mazzilli, Samuele Paparo Barbaro, Antonio Parisi, Salvatore Raffa, Nikki Wyrd. Special thanks to Francesca Zito for her impeccable work of transcription. Without the encouragement and assistance of Cafiero Franconi and the constant support of Anna Maria Del Signore and Ernesto Rossi this book would never have seen the light: they deserve a thank you from the bottom of my heart.

Giovanna Franconi
Internal Medicine
Department of Systems Medicine
Tor Vergata University of Rome, Rome
Italy

FURTHER READING

Cardini F *et al*. Clinical research in traditional medicine: priorities and methods. Complem Ther Med 2006; 14(4): 282–7.

CONSENT FOR PUBLICATION

Not applicable.

CONFLICT OF INTEREST

The author (editor) declares no conflict of interest, financial or otherwise.

ACKNOWLEDGEMENT

Declare none.

BIBLIOGRAPHY

[1] Unschuld PU, Tessenow H. Huang Di Nei Jing Su Wen An Annotated Translation of Huang Di's Inner Classic—Basic Questions University of California Press 2011.

[2] Van Nghi N. Huangdi Neijing Lingshu Books 1–3 with commentary Sugar Grove, NCJung Tao Productions 2005.

CHAPTER 1

Anatomy And Physiology of the Male Genital Tract

Abstract: The male genital tract consists of the testes, a ductal system and accessory glands. Sperm is produced in the testes and, combined with the fluids produced by the sex accessory organs, moves through the sperm ducts to reach the female reproductive tract. The chapter summarizes the anatomy and development of the male genital tract and the physiology of sperm production.

Keywords: Bulbourethral Glands, Epididymis, Follicle-Stimulating Hormone, FSH, GnRH, Kallman's Syndrome, Leydig Cells, LH, Luteinizing Hormone, prostate, Seminal Vescicles, Seminiferous Subules, Sertoli Cells, Sex Hormone Binding Globulin, Spermatids, Spermatogenesis, Spermatocytes, Spermatogonia, Steroidogenesis, Testosterone.

THE MALE GENITAL TRACT

The male genital tract has an external part, consisting of the penis and testicles, and an internal part, the sperm ducts (straight tubules, rete testis, efferent ducts, epididymis, vas deferens, ejaculatory duct and urethra) and the glands connected to the sperm ducts (seminal vesicles, bulbourethral glands and the prostate).

The male genital tract is shown schematically in Fig. (**1**).

The penis is the male organ of copulation, it wraps around the penile urethra and is used to deposit the semen into the vagina. It consists of three cylindrical masses of erectile tissue, namely the two corpora cavernosa, and the corpus spongiosum, which can fill with blood during sexual arousal.

The testes are a pair of ellipsoidal organs which measure about 5cm in length, 3cm in the anteroposterior direction and 3cm in width. They are mobile within the scrotal sac and their position is related to the relaxation or contraction of the cremaster and dartos muscles and of the wall of the scrotal sac. On palpation, their texture is hard-elastic. The tunica albuginea covers the testicles on the outside and deepens inwardly, outlining the septa. The septa divide the parenchyma into lobules, which consist of seminiferous tubules that are made up of germ cells, where spermatogenesis occurs. The terminal part of the tubules is straight (straight tubule) and ends in the rete testis, where the efferent ducts originate that reach the head of the epididymis. The epididymis adheres to the back of the testicle and may be compared to a storage area for sperm, which become mature and mobile during the transit from the head to the tail of the epididymis. During ejaculation the epididymis contraction allows the progression of sperm into the vas deferens and to the urethra. The vas deferens is about 30cm long and is formed of thick muscle tissue. It travels in the spermatic cord and goes through the inguinal canal to enter the pelvic cavity in a subperitoneal position; it passes laterally to the urinary bladder heading upwards, then it crosses the ureter and bends medially and posteriorly and, prior to entering the prostate, it enlarges and receives the excretory duct of the ipsilateral seminal vesicle; inside the prostate it continues as the ejaculatory duct and ends in the prostatic urethra.

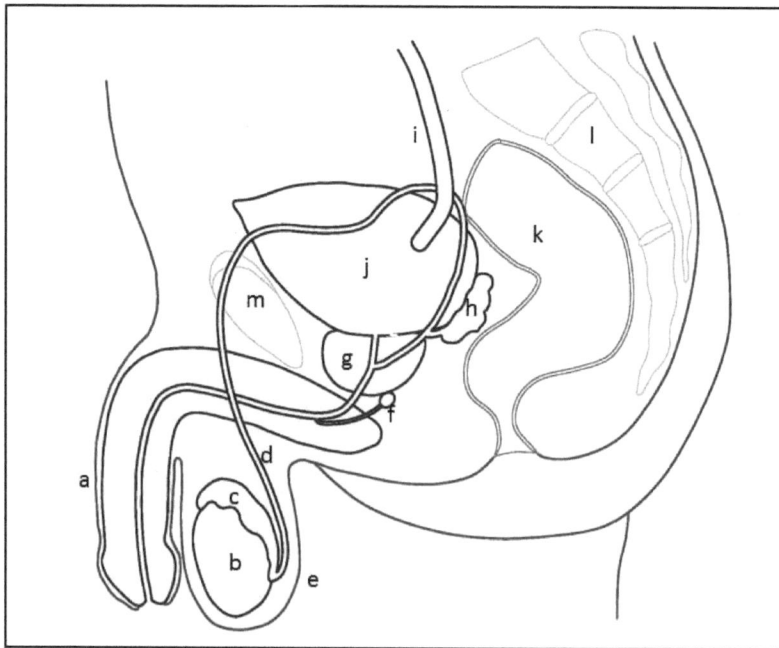

Fig. (1). Schematic representation of the male genital apparatus. a = penis; b = testis; c = epididymis; d = vas deferens; e = scrotal sac; f = bulbourethral gland (Cowper's gland); g = prostate; h = s eminal vesicle; i = ureter; j = urinary bladder; k = rectum; l = sacrum; m = pubic symphysis.

Spermatogenesis and steroidogenesis take place in the testes. Spermatogenesis includes all the processes involved in the production of male gametes, while steroidogenesis refers to the enzymatic reactions that lead to the production of male steroid hormones (androgens). Spermatogenesis and steroidogenesis occur in two compartments, which are morphologically and functionally different from each other: the tubular segment, consisting of seminiferous tubules, and the interstitial compartment, located between the seminiferous tubules. Although anatomically separated, both compartments are closely linked with each other and the integrity of both is required for sperm production of normal quantity and quality. These testicular functions are regulated by the hypothalamus and pituitary gland (endocrine regulation), and modulated by local testicular mechanisms (autocrine and paracrine factors).

The interstitial compartment represents about 15% of the total testicular volume, and besides connective tissue, blood and lymph vessels, nerve fibres, fibroblasts and immune cells, it contains the Leydig cells which produce testosterone. Leydig cells are activated during the first trimester of fetal life, and then at puberty to produce testicular androgens, and are influenced by luteinizing hormone (LH). In cases of inflammation, the macrophages and lymphocytes produce cytokines and other inflammatory substances.

The tubular compartment represents about 80% of the total testicular volume and contains the seminiferous tubules with germ cells and two different types of somatic cells, the peritubular cells and the Sertoli cells. This compartment is not vascularized, and is separated from the interstitial compartment by the lamina propria. Immediately below the lamina propria there are peritubular cells (myofibroblasts), that are involved in cell contractility and in the peristalsis of the seminiferous tubule. The contraction of these cells promotes the transport of mature sperm to the exit of the seminiferous tubules.

The testicular germ cells have a multi-layered arrangement. The cells close to the tubule basal lamina make up the pool of immature cells, which proliferate and begin the process of differentiation. The differentiation process happens within the tubule wall as the cells move toward the tubular lumen.

The Sertoli cells rest on the basement membrane and extend within the lumen of the seminiferous tubule for the entire thickness of the epithelial layer, supporting the orientation of the sperm during differentiation. In adulthood, these cells are mitotically inactive and account for about 35–40% of the volume of the tubular wall. They are responsible for the maturation of spermatozoa through their morphological and functional contact with sperm in the adult. Sertoli cells secrete cytokines, growth factors, opioid peptides, steroids, prostaglandins and modulators of cell division. One of their most important products is Anti-Müllerian hormone (AMH), which is secreted during the early stages of fetal life and determines the male phenotype. Until puberty, AMH is an index of testicular function, whilst after puberty its synthesis is inhibited by the increasing levels of testosterone. Other important products of Sertoli cells are inhibin and activins, which are secreted after puberty to regulate the secretion of FSH, and the androgen binding protein (ABP), which increases the concentration of testosterone in the seminiferous tubules to promote spermatogenesis. Sertoli cells also secrete tubular fluid, which maintains the patency of the lumen of the seminiferous tubule. The tubular fluid is not reabsorbed, thanks to the presence of the blood-testis barrier. This barrier is composed of the tight junctions between the Sertoli cells and it divides the seminiferous epithelium into two regions which are anatomically and functionally different. The immature germ cells are located in the basal region, while the subsequent stages of maturation are located in the region closer to the tubular lumen. The blood-testis barrier provides physical isolation for the haploid cells, which are antigenically different and thus avoid their recognition by the immune system (preventing autoimmune orchitis).

The accessory glands produce most of the liquid part of the seminal fluid. The seminal vesicles can be considered as glandular diverticula of the vas deferens. Their secretion, stimulated by the presence of androgens, is composed of alkaline fluid rich in proteins, sorbitol, fructose, citric acid and prostaglandins, and which constitutes about 60% of the volume of the seminal fluid.

The prostate is a glandular organ placed in the pelvis below the bladder. It has the shape, size and texture of a chestnut. It is surrounded by a dense fibrous capsule and is crossed by the ejaculatory ducts and prostatic urethra. The prostatic parenchyma consists of a set of tubulo-alveolar glands, surrounded by a fibrous tissue containing smooth muscle cells, which contract at the time of ejaculation. The prostate produces a slightly acidic and cloudy liquid, which constitutes 35% of the volume of the semen. The prostatic secretions contain acid phosphatase, amylase, proteases and other enzymes and prostaglandins, immunoglobulins, zinc and citric acid, to stimulate sperm motility.

The bulbourethral glands (or Cowper's glands) are small exocrine glands of 5–10 mm in diameter located at the root of the penis near the membranous urethra. They produce a fluid rich in glycoproteins and neutral sialoprotein, which facilitates the passage of sperm during ejaculation.

The composition of the seminal fluid and the origin of the different parts is shown in Table **1**.

DEVELOPMENT OF THE MALE GENITAL TRACT

Male sexual differentiation, like female sexual differentiation, occurs in three phases: the genetic sex determination initiated by genes encoded by the sex chromosomes, the gonadal sex determination (differentiation of the testes and the ovaries), and the phenotypic sex determination with development of the genital organs and the secondary sexual characteristics.

Table 1. Origin and characteristics of the different parts of the semen.

Origin	Volume	Comment
Bulbourethral glands	0.1–0.2 mL	Viscous, clear
Testes, epididymis	0.1–0.2 mL	Contains spermatozoa
Prostate	0.5–1.0 mL	Acidic, watery
Seminal vesicles	1.0–3.0 mL	Jelly-like, rich in fructose
Complete seminal fluid	2.0–5.0 mL	Liquefaction in 20–25 minutes

The process of sexual differentiation starts from the determination of the genetic sex, when at conception a pair of heterologous sex chromosomes (XY) is formed.

In the 46,XY embryo (male), gonads are undifferentiated and bipotential until the 6th week. Around the 7th–8th week of gestation gonadal sex determination begins. Several gene products, among which the most important are SRY (Sex Determining Region Y), SF-1 (Steroidogenic Factor 1), SOX-9 (SRY-related HMG box) and others, initiate the differentiation to the male gonad. SRY is located on the short arm of the Y chromosome and is the main determinant of testicular differentiation.

Phenotypic sex is based on the differentiation of internal and external genitalia during embryogenesis, and the subsequent appearance of secondary sexual characteristics at puberty. Around the 9th week of gestation Sertoli cells begin to produce AMH, which acts in a paracrine manner and promotes the apoptosis of Müllerian structures (which in females lead to the development of the uterus and fallopian tubes). Leydig cells begin to activate towards the 11th–17th week producing a high peak of circulating testosterone, which causes the masculinization of the internal genitalia. The masculinization of the external genitalia happens from the 14th week thanks to the crucial action of dihydrotestosterone (DHT), a hormone androgen derived from testosterone. DHT is involved in the differentiation of the Wolffian ducts (vas deferens, epididymis) of the urogenital sinus (prostate, urethra), and of the genital tubercle (glans and external genitalia). In the adult DHT acts as the primary androgen in the prostate, where it is responsible for benign prostate hypertrophy and contributes to the development of prostate cancer, while in the hair follicles DHT contributes to male pattern baldness.

TESTICULAR DESCENT

In the early stages of embryo life, testes are attached to the gonadal ridge in the posterior wall of the abdominal cavity. During fetal growth they descend to the pelvic cavity in an androgen-independent process. After the 26th week of gestation, the testes complete their descent into the scrotal sac in an androgen-dependent process. In 97% of infants the testicular descent is completed within the first 12 weeks of life. The presence of an abnormal position of the testicles is one of the most frequent congenital defects, and is associated with disorders of spermatogenesis and with an increased risk of developing testicular cancer.

HORMONAL CONTROL OF THE TESTICULAR FUNCTION

The male gonads are stimulated by gonadotropins (luteinizing hormone or LH and follicle-stimulating hormone or FSH), which control steroidogenesis and gametogenesis. LH and FSH are hormones synthesized by the anterior pituitary gonadotropic cells in both males and females, and in turn are regulated by the hypothalamic gonadotropin releasing hormone (GnRH, also called LHRH). The secretion of GnRH by the hypothalamic neurons occurs in a pulsatile manner, and is controlled by gonadal steroids and peptides and by adrenergic, dopaminergic, and endorphinic circuits, whose influence is both direct and *via* the hypothalamus. The reproductive axis is also regulated by metabolic signals, which detect the energy balance of the organism and, for example, are inhibited during prolonged fasting. Two forms of GnRH Have been identified, namely GnRH-I call (or GnRH) and GnRH-II, which are encoded by separate genes. The two forms are structurally very similar, but while GnRH-I regulates gonadotropins, GnRH-II acts as a neuromodulator and regulates sexual behaviour. GnRH-I is a decapeptide produced in the hypothalamic GnRH neurons, which originate from olfactory neurons. These neurons during embryonic development migrate to the olfactory bulb through the nasal septum in an extremely complex process that involves several genes. Alterations in these genes lead to Kallman's Syndrome, a form of hypogonadotropic hypogonadism associated with anosmia. The relationship between olfactory apparatus and hormones is exemplified by pheromones, substances responsible for stereotypical sexual and social behaviour. In humans, communication through smell seems to begin with puberty.

The gonadotropins LH and FSH are glycoprotein hormones secreted by the pituitary gland. They control the development, maturation and function of the gonad. LH and FSH are measurable in the pituitary gland as early as the 10th week of gestation, and during the 12th week in the peripheral blood. Testosterone is already produced by the fetal testis during the 10th week of gestation, under the stimulus of fetal LH and maternal human chorionic gonadotropin (hCG). This testosterone determines the initial phase of testicular migration and the development of male external genitalia. During childhood gonadotropin levels in the serum are very low, but at puberty there is a peak. FSH and LH exert their function through their specific receptors, and are negatively regulated (feedback) by gonadal steroid hormones.

Both testosterone (sperm maturation) and FSH (initiation of spermatogenesis) are potentially able to initiate and maintain spermatogenesis, but the combined action of LH, FSH, and testosterone is required to get a good effect on the quantitative production of sperm.

LH stimulates the Leydig cells and their production of testosterone. The concentration of testosterone within the testis is 80–100 times more than that in the peripheral blood; this means that a high amount of testosterone is needed for spermatogenesis. Men who abuse anabolic steroids or take exogenous testosterone have normal testosterone levels in their blood, but these are not sufficient to induce spermatogenesis, because at the same time the production of LH, which stimulates more production of intratesticular testosterone, is inhibited by peripheral androgens. This mechanism has been used to develop male contraception, because it is possible to suppress spermatogenesis in a normal man just with supplemental doses of testosterone which block the production of LH.

The regulation of testicular function is mainly under central control, but there are also several mechanisms of local control. These are of paracrine type (between adjacent cells), autocrine type (released from the cell and works on the same cell), and intracrine type (within the same cell). These local factors with modulating action are growth factors, immunological factors, and so on (see Table **2**).

Table 2. Local control of testicular function: Key factors produced in the testis that mediate intercellular communication in the control of testicular function and spermatogenesis.

Production site	Factors	Functions in the testis
Sertoli and Leydig cells	Transforming growth factor (TGF)-alfa	Growth stimulation
	TGF-beta	Growth inhibition, differentiation
	Insulin-like growth factor (IGF)-1	Homeostasis, DNA synthesis
	Interleuchin IL-1, IL-6	Regulation of growth of lymphocytes and other testicular cells, regulation of lymphocyte functions for immunological protection
	Fibroblast growth factor (FGF)	Growth stimulation
	Platelet-derived growth factor (PDGF)	Growth stimulation, differentiation

(Table 2) contd.....

Production site	Factors	Functions in the testis
Sertoli cells	Inhibin B	Correlates with spermatogenesis activity and sperm production
		Negative feedback on FSH secretion
	Estrogens	Proliferation, differentiation
	Stem cell factor (SCF)/ kit ligand (KL)	Growth stimulation in the primordial gonad (migration, proliferation and survival of primordial spermatogonia)
	Neurotrophines	Growth stimulation, migration, differentiation
	Glial-derived neurotrophic factor (GDNF)	Growth stimulation, differentiation
Leydig cells	Androgens	Differentiation
	Tumour necrosis factor (TNF)	Apoptosis, differentiation
Leukocytes	IL-1, IL-2, interferon (IFN)-gamma, tumour necrosis factor (TNF)-alfa	Regulation of steroidogenesis (Leydig cells)
		Inhibition of estradiol secretion (Sertoli cells)
Peritubular cells	Leukemia inhibitory factor (LIF)	Stimulation of fetal germ cell and Sertoli cell proliferation

Testosterone at the testicular level behaves as a paracrine factor; it is produced by Leydig cells, and acts on Sertoli cells. It is the main secretory product of the testis and is metabolized to 5alpha-dihydrotestosterone (DHT) by the testicular 5alpha-reductase and to estradiol by testicular aromatase. The active fraction of circulating testosterone is that not bound to transport proteins (albumin and Sex Hormone Binding Globulin - SHBG) and corresponds to approximately 2% of total testosterone. It is a local key regulator of spermatogenesis, although the relationship between concentrations of testicular testosterone and the production of germ cells is not yet completely clear. Testosterone and androgens regulate the hypothalamic-pituitary-testicular axis, are responsible for the development of the male phenotype during sexual differentiation, promote sexual maturation at puberty, regulate sexual behaviour, control bone physiology and the relationship between lean body mass and fat body mass.

Estradiol is produced in high quantities in men. The main part (60%) is of testicular origin after testosterone aromatization, while the rest comes from the adrenal cortex. Estrogens in the testis are also produced, during embryonic development, by Sertoli cells, while in adults they are synthesized by Leydig cells and by spermatids and spermatozoa. The concentration of estrogens at the level of the rete testis is very high, almost equal to that in women in the follicular phase. During fetal life the maternal alpha-fetoprotein blocks the influence of maternal estrogens on the fetus, while at birth the male experiences a spike in testosterone, which is called minipuberty. The brain of the newborn is imprinted in this stage, when testosterone is converted to estrogens, which have a critical role in the masculinization of the brain. Estrogens act especially on the neuronal circuits of sexual behaviour, whose signal will then be amplified by androgens to initiate sexual activity. Estrogens are used in a physiological way in the male resulting in a good reproductive function. Several experimental knock-out studies with abolition of estrogen receptors or aromatase have shown that estrogens have a very important role in spermatogenesis, steroidogenesis, and in male infertility.

Recently it has been discovered that Sertoli cells also have receptors for thyroid hormones, and many studies have now clarified that the thyroid gland significantly influences testicular development, spermatogenesis and male fertility. Hypothyroidism is associated with asthenozoospermia, decreased volume of ejaculate and alterations in sperm morphology; these alterations are reversible and are restored to normal when the euthyroid state is reached. Hyperthyroidism is associated with oligozoospermia and asthenozoospermia, and there is an improvement in sperm motility only after the treatment of thyroid abnormalities [1].

TESTICULAR TEMPERATURE

In men, testicular temperature is about 3–4° Celsius lower than the internal body temperature, since normal body temperature is incompatible with spermatogenesis. The cooling of the testis is ensured by several factors, in addition to the location in the scrotum outside of the body. The peculiar structure of the scrotal wall, which is corrugated and richly vascularized, allows for the loss of heat, and the arterio-venous pampiniform plexus permits the cooling of the arterial blood, as it enters the testis in physical proximity with the venous blood which comes from the testis and has a lower temperature. Exposure to heat may induce testicular germ cell apoptosis and sperm DNA damage through mechanisms of increased oxidative stress.

An increase in testicular temperature results in damage to the spermatogenesis, which can also become irreversible in the adult. In the case of a varicocele, which consists of an abnormal enlargement of the veins of the scrotum, scrotal temperature increases and can lead to problems with fertility in 40% of cases.

TESTICULAR IMMUNOLOGY

The gonocytes migrate to the testes during prenatal development, but spermatogonia begin to differentiate into spermatozoa only after puberty, when the immune system is already matured and systemic self-tolerance has developed. When spermatogonia proliferate and differentiate into spermatocytes, many new proteins are expressed on the surface, which are unknown to the immune system and this can stimulate immune reactions. The blood-testis barrier protects sperm maturation by creating an immunoprivileged site isolating the tubular content from the vascular compartment.

The immune privilege of the testis is given not only by the presence of the blood-testis barrier, but also depends on a specific regulation of the intratesticular immune function performed by testosterone, who has an immunosuppressive and immunomodulating role.

SPERMATOGENESIS

Spermatogenesis is a process that has many similarities with hematopoiesis. In both processes the stem cells (called germ cells in the testis) are capable of self-renewal and differentiation, providing a continuous production of functional cells. The normal testis of an adult man contains about one billion spermatozoa.

The germ cells develop and differentiate according to very specific processes. Primordial germ cells originate from the embryonic ectoderm in the 2nd gestational week, and by the 4th gestational week they migrate to the posterior wall of the abdominal cavity, where the primitive undifferentiated gonad develops. From the 7th gestational week the genes that stimulate the masculine differentiation of the undifferentiated gonad are activated by SRY. Germ cells become organized in testicular cords, which will become the seminiferous tubules at puberty, and Sertoli cells begin to produce AMH resulting in the involution of the paramesonephric ducts. Leydig cells differentiate around the 10th gestational week, and begin to produce testosterone under stimulation of maternal hCG and fetal LH. This causes the development of the internal genitalia, while the external genitalia develop from the 12th gestational week. At birth, the sharp fall in the blood concentration of maternal estrogens causes an increase in the infant male gonadotropins (mainly LH) and testosterone, which stimulate the proliferation of Sertoli cells and Leydig cells and the transformation of gonocytes into spermatogonia. Between the ages of 6 and 11 years there is a first maturation of the androgenic sexual characteristics in both sexes, stimulated by the adrenal androgens (adrenarche). At puberty the increase of pituitary LH stimulates testosterone production by the Leydig cells in the testes. This is converted into DHT, which is responsible for the development of the secondary sexual characteristics of the adolescent. A significant portion of testosterone is converted to estradiol, frequently responsible for a transient and modest gynecomastia.

Spermatogenesis is the process of sperm formation and involves more than 3,000 genes. Spermatozoa are highly specialized cells, consisting of a head and a flagellum. The head contains the nucleus, with a haploid set of chromosomes and very dense chromatin, and the acrosome, rich in lytic enzymes necessary for penetration into the ovum. The flagellum is very long, 50–60 microns, and has a sheath in the intermediate section composed of mitochondria, which provide energy for the movement of the flagellum itself.

Spermatogenesis can be divided into four phases:

1. Spermatogoniogenesis, which consists in the mitotic proliferation and differentiation of diploid germ cells (spermatogonia).
2. Meiotic division of the tetraploid germ cells (spermatocytes) with formation of haploid germ cells (spermatids); the round and elongated spermatids already contain all the information necessary for fertilization, and have been successfully used in ICSI (Intracytoplasmic Sperm Injection).
3. Spermiogenesis, which consists of the morphologic transformation of the spermatids into testicular spermatozoa.
4. Spermiation, resulting in the release of spermatozoa from the germinal epithelium into the tubular lumen.

Spermatogonia are diploid cells, which are located at the base of the seminiferous epithelium. There are three kinds of spermatogonia, type Ad (dark), type Ap (pale), and type B. Ad spermatogonia do not proliferate under normal circumstances and are considered testicular stem cells. They can, however, enter into mitosis when the total population of spermatogonia is drastically reduced, for example after extensive irradiation damage. In contrast, Ap spermatogonia can divide into two cells: one spermatogone Ap to replenish the pool of cells, and one spermatogone B that develops further. B spermatogonia begin to synthesize DNA and divide by mitosis, becoming tetraploid spermatocytes that go through the different stages of meiotic division. After the first meiosis they become secondary spermatocytes (with a haploid set of chromosomes), and after the second meiosis become spermatids. The prophase of the first meiosis lasts 1–3 weeks, while the other phases of the first meiosis and the whole second meiosis are completed within 1–2 days. The meiotic process is a critical event in gametogenesis, during which there is the complete recombination of genetic material, the reduction of the number of chromosomes and the development of spermatids.

Spermatids derived from the second meiotic division are inactive cells that must undergo a remarkable transformation (called spermiogenesis) to get to the final production of sperm. This transformation occurs in different parts of the cell:

• Condensation of the nucleus of the cell, which stabilizes the chromatin and helps to protect sperm DNA from mutagens.

- Formation of the acrosome, which is a structure that contains lytic enzymes that serve to penetrate the cumulus oophorus.
- Formation of the tail or flagellum, which includes the development and organization of the tubules, tubulin and dynein arms, and centrioles, which are important for sperm motility and for the cleavage of cells in the embryo.
- Expulsion of most of the cytoplasm.

During meiosis and spermiogenesis the cells are slowly pushed toward the lumen of the seminiferous tubule, while maintaining close contact with the Sertoli cells. The final release of spermatozoa into the tubular lumen is a process called spermiation and is very sensitive to hormonal, thermal and toxic influences.

The complex process of differentiation and proliferation of germ cells follows a precise time schedule and passes through several stages that are characterized by specific morphological criteria. For men the total duration of spermatogenesis is at least 64 days, or 74 days if the time for the renewal of spermatogonia is taken into account. The rate of maturation of sperm is hormone-independent, that is, once the process of differentiation starts it proceeds independently of the presence of hormones, while the amount of mature sperm is hormone-dependent.

The sperm from the seminiferous tubules that come along with the fluid secreted by the Sertoli cells go through the straight tubules in the cavities of the rete testis, from which they reach the epididymis. The epididymis maintains a unique microenvironment in which sperm may remain viable for more than two weeks, awaiting ejaculation, thanks to the presence of L-carnitine, myo-inositol, and glycerophosphocholine. In the proximal epididymis a further maturation of sperm takes place, enabling them to move.

During the process of ejaculation, sperm are detached from the distal portion of the tail of the epididymis and travel with the seminal fluid in order to fertilize the oocyte. Along the way, they must survive in the female tract, where capacitation occurs, and then must penetrate the lining of, and fuse with, the oocyte. Capacitation is a process that destabilizes the membrane of the sperm acrosome, making it more permeable and facilitating the acquisition of hyperactivated motility. In this way the capacitated sperm can penetrate the oocyte surface.

FURTHER READING

Hermo L, Robaire B. An Overview of Sperm Production. In: Carrell DT, Peterson CM, Eds. Reproductive Endocrinology and Infertility. Integrating Modern Clinical and Laboratory Practice. Springer 2010.

Nieschlag E, Behre HM, Nieschlag S. Andrology: Male Reproductive Health and

Dysfunction. Heidelberg, Germany: Springer 2010.

BIBLIOGRAPHY

[1]   La Vignera S, Vita R, Condorelli RA, *et al.* Impact of thyroid disease on testicular function. Endocrine 2017; 58(3): 397-407.
[http://dx.doi.org/10.1007/s12020-017-1303-8] [PMID: 28429281]

CHAPTER 2

Etiology and Pathogenesis of Male Infertility

Abstract: The causes of a reduced reproductive function (hypogonadism) may be classified according to the origin of the disease. Pre-testicular factors are due to alterations in the central regulation and the hypothalamic-pituitary-testis axis, while testicular factors (from primitive testicular alterations) manifest themselves as hypergonadotropic hypogonadism and are a major cause of azoospermia and oligozoospermia. When post-testicular factors are present, the reproductive and endocrine functions are normal but there is an obstacle to semen outflow because of occlusions, infections and inflammation of the genital tract. Genetic factors such as karyotype abnormalities, microdeletions of the Y chromosome mutations and polymorphisms are discussed extensively.

Keywords: Anejaculation, Anorchia, Cryptorchidism, Cystic Fibrosis, Endocrine Disruptor, Germinoma, Hypogonadism, Kallmann Syndrome, Klinefelter Syndrome, Laurence-Moon Syndrome, Lowe syndrome, Microdeletions of the Y Chromosome, Obstructive Azoospermia, Papillomavirus, polymorphism, Prader-Willi Syndrome, Retrograde Ejaculation, Robertsonian Translocation, Testicular Dysgenesis, Varicocele.

The function of the testes is both reproductive (spermatogenesis) and hormonal (steroidogenesis). There is hypogonadism when there is a deficiency in either the reproductive function, the endocrine function, or both. The causes of hypogonadism may be classified according to the origin of the disease, and can be testicular, pre-testicular or post-testicular. Mixed forms and genetic factors will be dealt with separately.

PRE-TESTICULAR FACTORS

In male infertility due to pre-testicular factors (due to alterations in the central regulation and the hypothalamic-pituitary-testis axis) both testicular functions, reproductive and endocrine, are typically affected. The causes of the pre-testicular forms are schematically shown in Table **3**.

Table 3. Pre-testicular causes of male infertility (about 10%).

Factors	Causes
Genetic	Kallmann syndrome
	Mutations of the GnRH receptor gene Mutations of the LH or FSH gene
Endocrine	Hypogonadotropic hypogonadism
	Hyperprolactinemia
	Hypopituitarism
	Congenital adrenal hyperplasia
	Thyroid dysfunction
	Hypercortisolism
Iatrogenic	Androgen intake
	Estrogen intake
	Doping

Hypogonadotropic Hypogonadism

Gonadal deficiency secondary to a central problem manifests itself as hypogonadotropic hypogonadism, where both reproductive and endocrine testicular functions are deficient in the presence of low levels of pituitary gonadotropins (FSH and LH). These forms may be congenital or acquired (see Table **4**).

Table 4. Classification of hypogonadotropic hypogonadism.

Congenital Forms	Hypothalamic (GnRH deficiency secondary to mutation of the GnRH gene) and pituitary (abnormal activity of GnRH or abnormal gonadotropin production secondary to mutation of GnRH receptor or mutation of FSH gene) causes
	Syndromic (associated with obesity, mental retardation, renal agenesis, *etc*) and nonsyndromic (isolated gonadotropin deficiency) forms
	Genetic disorders of gonadotropin secretion: Laurence-Moon-Biedl syndrome, Prader-Willy syndrome, Lowe syndrome, cerebellar ataxia
	Hemocromatosis

(Table 4) contd.....

Acquired Forms	Tumours (pituitary macroadenomas, craniopharyngiomas, hypothalamic tumours)
	Consequences of surgical treatment of pituitary tumours
	Vascular lesions (pituitary infarction, carotid aneurysm)
	Infiltrative disorders (sarcoidosis, histiocytosis, tuberculosis, fungal infections)
	Pituitary disorders: pituitary adenoma, empty sella syndrome
	Drug use: androgens, cyproterone, medroxyprogesterone acetate
	Drug abuse: anabolic steroids
	Endogenous hormone hyperproduction: adrenal tumours, Sertoli cell tumours, interstitial cell tumours of the testis, cirrhosis of the liver (these conditions can all produce estrogens); congenital adrenal hyperplasia; hyper- or hypo-thyroidism (hyperthyroidism alters the secretion of gonadotropins and increases the conversion of androgens into estrogens)

Idiopathic hypogonadotropic hypogonadism (IHH) is a form of isolated congenital hypogonadism, which is expressed during pre- and peri-pubertal ages because of a complete or partial defect of gonadotropin release. It is not associated with anatomical abnormalities of the hypothalamic-pituitary region. It may be associated with hypo- or anosmia in 60% of cases, and in this case it is named Kallmann syndrome. In the remaining 40% of cases there is normal olfactory sensitivity. The two forms are not separated from the etiopathogenic point of view.

Kallmann syndrome in males has a prevalence of 1:10,000. It is characterized by hypogonadotropic hypogonadism with anosmia or hyposmia. The anosmia is present only for the aromatic smells and there are no changes in sensitivity to irritant odours (*e.g.* ammonia) or to taste. A genetic defect is found more often in familial forms (50%) than in sporadic forms (10%). Kallmann syndrome consists of a hypothalamic GnRH deficiency secondary to a problem in the migration of hypothalamic GnRH neurons which originate from the olfactory neurons. The genes involved are mainly the KAL1 gene located on the X chromosome. KAL1 codes for a protein called anosmin, which is involved in the migration of olfactory and GnRH-secreting neurons during fetal life. Mutations of KAL1 are present in 15–50% of cases of Kallmann syndrome and may be accompanied by renal agenesis. Other genes involved in Kallmann syndrome are the FGFR1 (Fibroblast growth factor receptor 1), also known as KAL2, in 15% of cases; the gene that encodes the prokyneticin 2 (PROK2) and its receptor (PROKR2), in 10% of cases; and the CHD7 gene (chromodomain helicase DNA binding protein 7), in 7% of cases. Kallmann syndrome is often associated with renal abnormalities (unilateral or bilateral renal aplasia, horseshoe kidney), genital abnormalities (agenesis of the vas deferens), facial abnormalities (cleft lip, cleft palate), skin abnormalities (cafe au lait spots), or neurological manifestations as synkinesis, nystagmus, cerebellar ataxia, epilepsy, colour blindness, mental retardation, and so on.

In IHH GnRH-secreting neurons are localized correctly at the base of the hypothalamus but they are not activated. In this case anosmia will be absent. The genes involved are KISS1, GPR54 (G protein-coupled receptor 54), TAC3 (3 tachykinin or neurokinin B) and its receptor TACR3, and the gene of the GNRH receptor in case of resistance to GnRH.

While anosmia is typical of Kallmann syndrome, the clinical features of hypogonadism are present in both forms and depend on the age of onset. If hypogonadism develops in the prepubertal child, the testes are small and often cryptorchid, the prostate is small, libido is absent, body proportions are eunuchoid and the secondary sexual characteristics are absent. Without androgen treatment these men have little or no sexual activity and present with aspermia or azoospermia. Early osteoporosis can develop. If hypogonadism develops in the postpubertal male, the phenotype is variable. In general, the penis and testicles are normal, but the prostate becomes smaller, libido decreases, and there is a decrease in ejaculate volume and spermatogenesis. There may be weakness and muscle wasting, anemia and osteoporosis.

The first-level tests for the diagnosis of hypogonadism are the spermiogram for the evaluation of the gametogenic function, and the dosage of total testosterone for the evaluation of the steroidogenic function. The assessment of free testosterone is appropriate only if the total testosterone levels are lower than normal, but not obviously pathological. The diagnosis of hypogonadism is made after finding low levels of testosterone.

The GnRH stimulation test will result in a response only after a period of "priming" with pulsatile GnRH. It helps to differentiate the pituitary forms from the hypothalamic forms. Other second-level diagnostic tests include magnetic resonance imaging of the hypothalamic-pituitary region (to assess the olfactory bulbs, and to reveal any cancer), renal ultrasound (for renal agenesis), bone densitometry and semen analysis.

Other Congenital Hypogonadotropic Hypogonadisms

There are some rare genetic disorders that cause hypogonadotropic hypogonadism.

Laurence-Moon syndrome is a rare genetic autosomal recessive disorder, in which hypogonadotropic hypogonadism is associated with mental retardation, retinitis pigmentosa, and spastic paraplegia.

Prader-Willi syndrome arises from a partial deletion of chromosome 15 (15q11–q13 deletion of the region) and is characterized by hypogonadism, short stature, obesity, hypotonia and mild mental retardation.

Lowe syndrome—or oculo-cerebro-renal syndrome—is a rare X-linked disorder, associated with hypogonadism and congenital cataracts, Fanconi type proximal renal tubulopathy, hypotonia, areflexia and mental retardation.

Hypogonadism can also be associated with cerebellar ataxia in a rare autosomal recessive syndrome characterized also by dementia, deafness, peripheral neuropathy, and corticospinal signs.

Hyperprolactinemia

The presence of hyperprolactinemia may be responsible for both reproductive and sexual dysfunctions. Common symptoms in patients with prolactin-secreting pituitary tumours are loss of libido, impotence, gynecomastia and galactorrhea. Hyperprolactinemia may also be secondary to the use of drugs such as amitriptyline, imipramine, butyrophenones, phenothiazines, sulpiride, pimozide, methadone, amphetamine, morphine, estrogens, metoclopramide, methyldopa, and reserpine.

Hyperprolactinemia may be the cause of infertility in about 11% males with oligozoospermia. It inhibits the pulsatile secretion of GnRH causing secondary hypogonadism, and it also influences directly spermatogenesis and steroidogenesis by acting on receptors in Sertoli cells and Leydig cells in the testes, causing primary hypogonadism and infertility.

Hyperprolactinemia is one of the reversible causes of infertility. Medical therapy with bromocriptine or cabergoline normalizes serum prolactin levels, and restores the gonadal function.

Androgen Abuse

A normal spermatogenesis requires high levels of intratesticular testosterone to support spermatogenesis and inhibit germ cells apoptosis. The exogenous administration of androgens suppresses the production of GnRH from the hypothalamus and of gonadotropins from the pituitary, thereby reducing the concentration of intratesticular testosterone.

Professional athletes sometimes abuse anabolic androgenic substances as an ergogenic aid to improve muscle mass and strength, at doses up to 40 times higher than the physiological replacement therapy. Anabolic steroids are also abused by members of the general population to improve body image. In the United States,

4–6% of high school males admit to using these substances. Despite high doses of serum androgens, all of exogenous origin, intratesticular concentrations are often not sufficient to maintain a normal spermatogenesis resulting in hypogonadotropic hypogonadism, testicular atrophy, and azoospermia. The abuse of anabolic steroids should be suspected in muscular men with normal libido, normal erectile function, testicular atrophy, infertility, and low levels of gonadotropins and testosterone. Fertility is usually restored within four months after discontinuation of androgen, but hypogonadotropic hypogonadism may persist for up to three years. If seminal and hormonal recovery does not occur, after six months it is possible to start a treatment with gonadotropins to stimulate spermatogenesis.

There is no indication for androgen therapy in male infertility. On the contrary, the use of exogenous androgens is rather effective for male contraception.

TESTICULAR FACTORS

In male infertility due to testicular factors (from primitive testicular alterations) often only the reproductive function is affected. The causes of the testicular forms are schematically shown in Table **5**.

Table 5. Testicular causes of male infertility (about 75%).

Factors	Causes
Congenital	Anorchia
	Cryptorchidism
Genetic	Chromosomic abnormalities: Klinefelter syndrome, translocations, duplications and partial deletions
	Genic abnormalities: androgen insensitivity syndrome and Y chromosome microdeletions
Acquired	Testicular trauma
	Testicular torsion
	Urogenital tract infections
	Sexually transmitted diseases
	Iatrogenic (surgery, chemotherapy, radiotherapy, drugs which inhibit testosterone synthesis and action)
	Heat
	Testicular cancer
	Varicocele
	Systemic diseases (liver cirrhosis, renal failure)
	Lifestyle (smoke, alcohol, *etc.*)
Idiopathic	(Not known)

The testicular forms of male infertility manifest themselves as hypergonadotropic hypogonadism and are a major cause of azoospermia and oligozoospermia. Several different specific testicular pathologies have been described, but the idiopathic form is the most frequent. Often idiopathic infertility is linked to genetic causes.

Cryptorchidism

Cryptorchidism corresponds to undescended testicle(s) at birth. It is a very common abnormality of the urogenital system (3–5% of males born at term). The testis that is undescended at birth can descend spontaneously within the first year of age. If such an event does not happen, medical (hormonal) intervention and/or surgical intervention (orchidopexy) are needed to facilitate the descent and preserve the reproductive capacity. Therapeutic intervention should be carried out within the second year of life, because cryptorchidism is a risk factor for abnormalities of spermatogenesis and for an increase in incidence of germ cell cancer of the testis. Males with bilateral cryptorchidism have a higher incidence of fertility problems in adulthood compared to males with unilateral cryptorchidism. These percentages will be reduced if cryptorchidism is treated promptly. Men with a medical history of undescended testes should check periodically both the spermiogram and the ultrasound examination of the testicles from puberty.

Testicular Tumours and Testicular Dysgenesis

Testicular cancer is a rare disease and at the same time the most common malignancy in males between 15 and 35 years of age. Its incidence is increasing, mainly in industrialized countries. The main risk factor is cryptorchidism, followed by family history and by factors related to intrauterine life, such as maternal exposure to alcohol, sedatives and ionizing radiation. Exposure to environmental factors is also important, as it is more common in crude oil and agriculture workers.

In the majority of cases (>90%) testicular tumours originate from the germinal epithelium of the seminiferous tubules (germinoma). It manifests itself as a painless testicular mass or testicular swelling. In the presence of a testicular mass, the examination of first choice is testicular ultrasonography with colour Doppler, which allows differentiation of a benign from a malignant process with high specificity and sensitivity. The specific tumour markers for testicular tumours are beta human chorionic gonadotropin (beta-hCG), alpha-fetoprotein (AFP), carcinoembryonic antigen (CEA), lactate dehydrogenase (LDH), neuron-specific enolase (NSE) and placental alkaline phosphatase (PLAP).

Testicular cancer can adversely affect fertility either indirectly, due to the therapies used for its treatment (chemotherapy and radiotherapy), or directly. In fact, testicular cancer is epidemiologically linked to infertility, cryptorchidism and hypospadias, constituting a syndrome called "testicular dysgenesis". This means that infertile men have an increased risk of developing testicular tumours, up to 2.8 times more than the general population. At the base of testicular dysgenesis there would be a disturbance of the maturation of Sertoli cells, which would result in a reduction of germ cell differentiation, resulting in infertility and increased risk of testicular cancer; at the same time a disturbance of the maturation of Leydig cells would lead to a deficiency of testosterone, resulting in hypospadias and cryptorchidism, two diseases that are typically affected by androgen levels. The etiology of testicular dysgenesis is not linked to genetic factors, because the genetic background of the people involved has remained the same while there has been an increased incidence of testicular dysgenesis in the last 50 years. Probably the etiology is linked to environmental factors, such as increased exposure to endocrine disruptors [1].

Endocrine Disruptors

The decline in sperm quality and the simultaneous increase in the incidence of testicular cancer, cryptorchidism and hypospadias have a regional variation, suggesting an association with environmental factors such as exposure to endocrine disruptors [2].

According to the definition of the European Union; "an endocrine disruptor is an exogenous substance or mixture that alters the function of the endocrine system, causing adverse effects on the health of an organism, or its progeny, or of a (sub) population." Endocrine disruptors are heterogeneous compounds which have the ability to modify various endocrine mechanisms, either by mimicking natural hormones, or by inhibiting their action and/or altering the normal regulatory function of the endocrine systems. The endocrine disruptors have many possible routes of exposure with risk of additive or synergistic effects and/or the possibility of effects at very low doses. They mainly affect the reproductive system and the thyroid gland, especially in the early stages of pre-and postnatal development, inducing a spectrum of effects which an increasing number of studies associate with chronic-degenerative and metabolic diseases and infertility.

According to their use in agriculture and in everyday life, endocrine disruptors can be separated into chemical categories that include pesticides, industrial chemicals, phyto-hormones, *etc*. Table **6** lists the main endocrine disruptors acting on the reproductive system. Among the listed compounds, phytoestrogens are those probably most extensively in contact with the general population.

Table 6. Main endocrine disruptors acting on the reproductive system.

Categories	Active compounds	Actions on the endocrine system
Persistent organic contaminants	DDT, DDE (DDT metabolite) (insecticides)	Estrogenic agonist (DDT); androgenic antagonist (DDE); also thyreostatic effects
	Dioxins and dioxin-like compounds (byproducts of combustion processes)	Aryl hydrocarbon receptor agonists and progesterone receptor agonists with complex endocrine effects; carcinogenic effects
	Hexachlorobenzene (industrial compound and biocide)	Interference with glucose and lipid metabolism; thyreostatic effects
	Polychlorobiphenyls	Complex effects on endocrine, nervous and immune systems, interference with steroid hormones
	Cadmium	Estrogenic agonist
	Arsenic	Interference with glucocorticoid receptor; increase of oxidative stress
Compounds utilized in:	Azoles (fungicides)	Steroid synthesis inhibition; specific aromatase inhibitors
	Organochlorides (endosulfan, methoxychlor)	Estrogenic and antiandrogenic effects
	Linuron (herbicide)	Androgen receptor antagonist
	Procymidone (fungicide)	Androgen receptor antagonist
Industrial compounds	Alkylphenols (byproducts of industrial detergents)	Estrogenic agonists
	Bisphenol A (polycarbonates in baby feeding bottles, plastic containers, pipes for drinking water; epoxy resins in aluminum can coatings, coating for wine and water bottles; materials for dental amalgams)	α estrogen receptor agonist, possible effects on thyroid gland
	Phthalates (PVC plastics, excipients for glues, air fresheners, cosmetics, inks)	Estrogenic/antiandrogenic effects
	Perfluoro-octanes (coating of non-stick pans, sportswear, Gore-Tex, additives of glues, cosmetics, insecticides; high power of bioaccumulation)	Neurobehavioral effects, likely to interfere with the hypothalamic-pituitary axis and thyroid gland
Phytoestrogens	Genistein (in soy-based supplements, including infant formulas)	Selective modulation of α and β estrogen receptors
	Lignans (many plant foods)	Selective modulation of α and β estrogen receptors
	Zearalenone (contamination of feed)	Selective modulation of α estrogen receptor

The vast majority of endocrine disruptors do not induce gene mutations, but act on the epigenome during fetal and perinatal life, causing diseases in adulthood [3]. In addition to reduced fertility, endocrine disruptors may be responsible for prostate and testicular cancer, abnormal sexual development, disorders of the pituitary and thyroid gland, immune suppression, and neurobehavioral effects. The genetic consequences of exposure to endocrine disruptors could be transmitted for several generations.

Endocrine disruptors implicated at the biological level are oxidative stress, which alters sperm function by increasing free radicals and cytokines in the testis, and heat, which increases free radicals in the testis, reduces testosterone biosynthesis, alters spermatogenesis, and damages the testis.

The endocrine disruptors implicated at the pharmacological level are chemotherapy and radiation therapy, which may result in alterations of spermatogenesis up to total sterility, and drugs which may act on different stages of sperm maturation. Chemotherapy affects directly the germinal epithelium and Sertoli cells with direct toxic effects in a dose-dependent manner. The most gonadotoxic chemotherapeutic agents are the alkylating agents, the antimetabolites, and the vinca alkaloids, while the least gonadotoxic are methotrexate, cisplatin and 6-mercaptopurine. The germinal epithelium appears to be more resistant to toxic drugs before puberty than in adulthood, but is particularly sensitive to radiation, while the Leydig cells are relatively radioresistant. The damage to germ cells is reversible for exposures below 600 rad. Above this level it is likely that the damage is permanent.

The recovery of spermatogenesis after chemotherapy or radiotherapy may take up to 2–3 years, even in men receiving low doses of radiation, but sometimes the damage is irreversible. It is thus very important, whenever and wherever possible, to freeze the sperm (cryopreservation) before any such treatment begins.

Table **7** lists other pharmacological agents with spermatotoxic activity or acting on.

Table 7. Actions of drugs and narcotics on spermatogenesis.

Action on fertility	Drugs
Direct spermatozoon's	Cimetidine, sulfasalazine, antihistamines, nitrofurantoin, ethanol, marijuana
Decrease of spermatic motility	Antidepressants, antibiotics chlorpromazine, diazepam, local anesthetics, propranolol
Abnormal synthesis of testosterone	Cyproterone, alcohol, ketoconazole, spironolactone

(Table 7) contd.....

Action on fertility	Drugs
Testosterone antagonism	Cimetidine
Secondary hypogonadism	Marijuana, heroin, methadone

Varicocele

Varicocele is an enlargement of the venous system of the testis, either secondary to obstructed venous outflow, or more frequently idiopathic in nature. The presence of varicosities of the pampiniform plexus, which drains the blood from the testis, causes an environmental condition which is unfavourable for normal spermatogenesis. This is probably due to the rise of the testis temperature (due to venous stasis), to the retrograde flow of toxic metabolites through the incontinent vein, or to the blood stagnation with hypoxia of the germinal epithelium.

Varicocele occurs predominantly at puberty and worsens clinically with age. It affects most frequently the left testicle (95%) and rarely the right testicle (5%), due to the different anatomical features of the two venous systems. It has an incidence of 10–20% in the general male population and is present in 30–40% of men with fertility problems. About 50% of men with varicocele have poor semen quality. It is important that varicocele be diagnosed early in adolescence, because in some men it can cause a progressive reproductive damage, regardless of its size, with alterations in sperm number, motility and morphology.

The diagnosis of varicocele is based on the physical and ultrasound examination of male genitalia. Based on the physical exam it can be classified into subclinical varicocele, in which the varicocele is not palpable or visible at rest or during the Valsalva maneuver but detectable only with instrumental methods; Grade I, in which the varicocele is palpable only during the Valsalva maneuver; Grade II, in which the varicocele is palpable but not visible at rest; Grade III, in which the varicocele is visible and palpable at rest.

Table **8** lists the classification of varicocele according to Doppler ultrasound findings.

Table 8. Classification of varicocele with colour Doppler ultrasound investigation.

GRADE	ECHOGRAPHIC FINDINGS
1	Prolonged inguinal reflux only during Valsalva maneuver
2	Small posterior varicosity with sovra-testicular reflux only during Valsalva maneuver
3	Varicosity only when standing, sovra- and peri-testicular reflux only during Valsalva maneuver

(Table 8) contd.....

GRADE	ECHOGRAPHIC FINDINGS
4	Peri-testicular reflux at rest which increases when standing and during Valsalva maneuver (usually associated to testicular hypotrophy)
5	Clear venous ectasia when standing, peri-testicular reflux at rest which does not increase with Valsalva maneuver

There is no consensus about what the indications are for surgical or radiological correction of varicocele. There is evidence that the semen parameters may improve after correction of varicocele only in the presence of clinical varicocele, in a window which is between 6 and 12 months after surgery. Surgical treatment of varicocele is generally recommended in the following cases:

• Man with palpable varicocele, couple with established infertility, the female partner has normal fertility or a potentially treatable causes of infertility, and the man has abnormal semen analysis parameters.
• Man with palpable varicocele, abnormal semen analysis and the desire for future fatherhood.
• Adolescents with objective evidence of reduced testicular volume by the side of the varicocele (in case of bilateral varicocele and testicular hypotrophy or atrophy, it is necessary to perform other diagnostic tests).
• Symptomatic varicocele.

Treatment can be surgical, with open or laparoscopic or microsurgical methods, or it may use techniques of interventional radiology with embolization or sclerotherapy of the scrotal-testicular veins. Treatment complications consist mainly of persistence or recurrence of varicocele (9–45%) and hydrocele (10%).

In cases of normozoospermia and subclinical varicocele, there is no benefit of treatment *versus* clinical observation. It is advisable to perform genetic screening in the infertile males with varicocele, because varicocelectomy in the presence of genetic abnormalities will not improve fertility.

Sexually Transmitted Diseases

Sexually transmitted diseases (STDs) are infectious diseases that are very common in people with risky sexual behaviour. The mode of transmission is mainly by direct infection during sexual activities without protection (without a condom). The infection may also occur through oral sex. STDs have a significant role for public health due to their high incidence, the high proportion of asymptomatic or mild illness that promotes the spread of these infections, and the complications such as chronicization, male and female infertility, neoplastic transformation, and synergy with HIV infection.

In men, the STDs that can cause infertility are Neisseria *gonorrhoeae* and HIV, while the role of Chlamydia trachomatis, Ureaplasma urealyticum, Genital Herpes (Herpes simplex, HSV), and Trichomonas vaginalis is not certain. STDs affect male fertility because they can directly affect the reproductive organs with localized infections (orchitis, prostatitis, epididymitis) and/or stenosis of the urethra, of the vas deferens and of the tubules, or because they can cause systemic diseases that weaken the efficiency of the reproductive system.

Human papillomavirus (HPV) infection in men has been given little attention because it has been linked only to genital warts; while it is the causative agent of cervical cancer in women, the infected man was simply considered a carrier of the HPV infection for women. However, the incidence of male cancers from HPV (penile cancer, anal cancer, and cancer of the head and neck) is increasing, especially in homosexuals and immunocompromised individuals, and when HPV is present in the seminal fluid it may have an important role in male infertility. In fact, HPV alters the characteristics of sperm and may cause the failure of assisted reproductive techniques. HPV infection in men is often asymptomatic, and should be suspected when there are HPV-related warts, when the partner is HPV-positive or has recurrent miscarriages, or if the man has had several sexual partners or if he is immunocompromised or has idiopathic asthenozoospermia.

Testicular Torsion

The testicular torsion is a rotation of the testicle around its vascular axis; it is characterised by a rapid onset of acute pain and swelling of the testicle and must be treated promptly (within a few hours from the onset) to avoid irreversible vascular damage to the testicle.

Surgery

A temporary suppression of spermatogenesis, which may last for 2–6 months, may occur after any surgery, especially if it has been done under general anesthesia. If the surgery has been performed in the abdomen or pelvis (bladder, colon, prostate, *etc.*), spermatogenesis may be suppressed in an irreversible way.

Lifestyle

Smoking may decrease the reproductive capacity of men and women, acting both at a local and a systemic level. Smoke crosses the blood-testis barrier and can affect all semen parameters, in particular causing asthenozoospermia and teratozoospermia, can cause damage to sperm DNA from oxidative stress and may reduce the success of assisted reproductive techniques. At the systemic level smoking can alter the hypothalamic-pituitary axis through the stimulation of the release of GH, cortisol, vasopressin and oxytocin, which in turn inhibit the release of LH. The effects of smoking, however, seem to affect only susceptible individuals, because smokers as a group do not show a reduction in fertility. However, males with low sperm quality could benefit from smoking cessation. Tobacco smoke contains a number of mutagens which may affect the offspring, even when it is the father who is smoking, so smoking cessation might be beneficial also for the health of the unborn child.

Habitual alcohol intake of at least five units/week negatively affects sperm concentration and morphology, and the effect is more apparent for men with a habitual alcohol intake above 25 units/week. One unit of alcohol is 10 mL of pure alcohol, which corresponds roughly to a small glass of wine, half a pint of beer or a single measure of liquor. Alcohol may have a direct spermatotoxic effect, or alcohol consumption may be associated with other health behaviours which negatively affect spermatogenesis [4].

Sperm cells have receptors for cannabinoids (CB1 and CB2), and marijuana use can adversely affect sperm motility and testosterone levels. Cocaine use has been associated with oligozoospermia.

The increase in scrotal temperature has a close correlation with sperm quality. Occupational exposure to heat has been associated with alterations in sperm quality, while sitting in a sedentary job and wearing tight underwear, which may lead to an increase in scrotal temperature, do not have a large impact on male fertility. However, any factor that prevents a normal cooling of the testicle can lead to an adverse effect on spermatogenesis, so men who have sperm abnormalities, in particular in number and motility, should be advised on how to minimize scrotal overheating, because small changes in lifestyle can have beneficial effects on spermatogenesis.

POST-TESTICULAR FACTORS

In male infertility due to post-testicular factors, the reproductive and endocrine functions are normal but there is an obstacle to semen outflow because of occlusions, infections and inflammation of the genital tract. The causes of the post-testicular forms are schematically shown in Table **9**.

Table 9. Post-testicular causes of male infertility (about 15%).

Factors	Causes
Genetic	CFTR gene mutation

(Table 9) contd.....

Factors	Causes
Acquired obstruction of the seminal ducts	Postinfectious
	Iatrogenic
	Autoimmunity
Ejaculation disorders	Retrograde ejaculation (diabetes, iatrogenic)
	Anejaculation
	Severe erectile dysfunction
Malformations of penis and urethra	Hypospadias

Obstructive Azoospermia

Azoospermia, defined as the complete absence of sperm in the semen, is present in less than 2% of all men, and in 15% of infertile men. Although there may be many causes of azoospermia, the obstruction of the ductal system is responsible for about 40% of cases. The obstruction may be at the level of the epididymis, the vas deferens or the ejaculatory duct. The most frequent causes are vasectomy, the consequences of serious infections, genito-urinary obstructions that caused scarring, and iatrogenic injury during surgical procedures in the groin or scrotum, even during varicocelectomy. Among the congenital anomalies of the ducts the best known is cystic fibrosis, which will be described in the chapter on genetic diseases. Another congenital anomaly, more common than cystic fibrosis, is Young's syndrome, also associated with lung bronchiectasis. In Young's syndrome the ultrastructure of the cilia is normal and there is no pancreatic involvement, but the body of the epididymis is obstructed by thick secretions, preventing the passage of sperm.

There may be functional distal obstructions from neurogenic, psychogenic and pharmacological causes that result in azoospermia, cryptozoospermia, or severe OAT (Oligozoospermia, Asthenozoospermia and Teratozoospermia). The neurogenic causes are comparable to a localized neuropathy (achalasia like) and may be found in juvenile diabetes, multiple sclerosis, in polycystic kidney disease and in the outcome of pelvic surgery. These damage the peristalsis of the vas deferens with a consequent lack of emission and/or problems in the closure of the bladder neck at the time of ejaculation. The psychogenic anejaculation is generally accompanied by anorgasmia and should be distinguished from anejaculation secondary to dysfunction of the central or peripheral nervous system. The drugs involved in the functional obstruction are antihypertensives, antidepressants, antipsychotics and alcohol.

Retrograde Ejaculation

Retrograde ejaculation occurs during orgasm when seminal fluid is not released into the penile urethra but into the bladder. The main causes of retrograde ejaculation are classified into three groups: anatomic causes (after bladder neck surgery or because of a congenital problem), neurological causes (diabetic neuropathy, lesions of the spinal cord, multiple sclerosis, or damage during retroperitoneal surgery), and pharmacological causes (paralysis of the bladder neck by drugs such as alpha blockers, antidepressants and antipsychotics). Diagnosis is done after the recovery of semen and/or sperm in a urine sample obtained immediately after orgasm.

Antisperm Antibodies

Data from the literature suggest that 8–10% infertile males have an autoimmune reaction to sperm that can interfere with fertility. The presence of antisperm antibodies (ASA) can alter sperm motility and concentration, and can be responsible for the presence of areas of sperm agglutination. ASA may interfere with the penetration of sperm in the cervical mucus, and with the membrane receptors involved in the sperm-oocyte interaction during embryonic development, and may cross-react with embryonic antigens to block implantation. Fertilization decreases with increasing intensity of the autoimmune phenomenon. The presence of high antibody titers occur in the absence of specific symptoms, therefore the assessment of immunological infertility is based solely on laboratory diagnostics.

MIXED FORMS

There are mixed forms of male infertility in which abnormalities are present simultaneously at multiple levels of the hypothalamic-pituitary-testis axis.

Obesity

Obesity and being overweight are associated with an increased incidence of male infertility. A BMI greater than 25 is associated with a 25% reduction in the number and motility of sperm. Obese men often have increased scrotal temperature, decreased libido, increased sperm DNA fragmentation, and hormonal imbalances that lead to infertility. In particular, obese men have lower serum testosterone levels proportional to the degree of obesity and an increase in circulating estrogens which suppress testosterone synthesis through the modulation of the hypothalamic-pituitary-testicular axis. This is due to the adipose mass which expresses high levels of aromatase, the enzyme which converts testosterone into estradiol. In these men the suppression of estradiol by aromatase inhibitors may lead to an improvement in sperm quality. Obesity can also directly reduce the number of Sertoli cells [1].

Paternal Age

The age of the father, especially when above 40 years, is directly proportional to abortivity. With increasing paternal age, the risks for the offspring are related to the presence of chromosomal abnormalities, which are found in 35% of spontaneous abortions (*e.g.*, trisomy 16), in 4% of stillbirths, and in 0.3% of live births (in particular triple X, trisomy 13, trisomy 18, and trisomy 21). Paternal age contributes also to trisomy 21 (Down syndrome) when the female partner is more than 40 years of age. In this case the paternal contribution is about 50% [5].

Sex chromosome abnormalities are more frequent in the sperm of older men, who are more likely to produce aneuploid gametes.

The influence of paternal age in congenital malformations in the offspring has been documented for gastroschisis, omphalocele, spina bifida and orofacial and heart malformations.

Systemic Diseases

Many diseases can induce alterations in the number and quality of sperm both because of a direct action on the hormonal balance, and indirectly because of the drugs used to treat them.

The end-stage renal failure in males is associated with decreased libido, impotence, gynecomastia and impaired spermatogenesis. Gonadotropins are elevated and testosterone levels are decreased. The cause of hypogonadism in uremia is probably multifactorial: serum levels of prolactin are elevated in 25% of patients, and there is an excess of estrogens. The uremic hypogonadism improves after kidney transplantation.

Many men with liver cirrhosis also have testicular atrophy, impotence and gynecomastia. Testosterone levels are decreased, whereas estradiol is increased as a result of increased peripheral conversion of testosterone to estrogen. LH and FSH levels are only moderately elevated compared with the low levels of serum testosterone.

Hypogonadism is present also in many men with sickle cell disease. Although gonadotropin levels can be variable, testosterone levels are low. Hypogonadism in sickle cell anemia is probably secondary to a combination of testicular and hypothalamic-pituitary causes.

Fever may affect spermatogenesis, either directly or for the use of antibiotics given to treat the underlying disease. If it exceeds 38.5°C it can affect spermatogenesis for 2–6 months.

Hemochromatosis

About 80% of men with hemochromatosis have testicular dysfunction. Hypogonadism can be primary because of the deposition of iron in the testes, but can also be secondary because of iron deposition in the pituitary gland.

GENETIC FACTORS

Sperm formation takes place in a sequential manner (mitosis, meiosis, and postmeiotic differentiation), and each phase is controlled by a complex genetic program. This genetic program also controls other correlated physiological processes, such as the regulation of the hypothalamus-pituitary-gonadal axis and the development and differentiation of germ cells. It is estimated that approximately 10% of human genes are involved in spermatogenesis, but only about 96 genes involved in spermatogenesis have been partially elucidated, in addition to the genes contained in the Y chromosome [6].

Somatic cells and spermatogonia have a set of diploid chromosomes (2n = 46), while the chromosomal set deriving from the first meiotic division consists of 23 chromosomes (haploid). The haploid human genome is composed of three billion base pairs, of which only about 1% consists of coding sequences, and contains 25,000–30,000 genes. A portion of the genetic code of humans is located in the mitochondria (mitochondrial genome).

The main genetic alterations involved in male infertility known to date are:

- Karyotype abnormalities.
- Microdeletions of the Y chromosome.
- Polymorphisms correlated to risk factors and to new candidate genes.
- Mutations in the androgen receptor gene.
- Mutations in candidate genes for central hypogonadism.
- Alterations in the CFTR gene.

Genetic factors are believed to be responsible of infertility in about 15–30% of infertile males. In addition to strictly genetic factors, the interaction between genes and environment or epigenetic factors may play a role in some cases of idiopathic male infertility, especially in different populations or individual susceptibility to endocrine disruptors. Epigenetic factors are non-genetic factors that cause a different expression of the genes: what changes is the phenotype, but the DNA does not change. This may happen through mechanisms that include DNA methylation, histone acetylation, chromatin remodelling, gene silencing, and so on. These processes alter the physical accessibility to the regions of the genome and thus gene expression. Epigenetic changes are preserved when cells divide, and if they are present in a sperm or an oocyte that is fertilized, they can be inherited by the next generation.

The presence of a genetic disease affects the reproductive capacity at different levels, generally resulting in a reduction in the number and motility of sperm. It is important to diagnose the presence of genetic disease to preserve the reproductive capacity and to generate a healthy fetus.

Karyotype Abnormalities

The karyotype is the "chromosome formula", that is, the analysis of the number of chromosomes, their size, the position of the centromere, the banding pattern (karyogram), and their aberrations (deletions, duplications, translocations, inversions, insertions, *etc.*).

Conventional cytogenetics examines chromosomes during metaphase, when they have the highest condensation and are best detected. Molecular cytogenetics uses molecular genetics techniques to achieve a higher resolution. Fluorescence In Situ Hybridization (FISH) is the basic method of molecular cytogenetics, and can be used to study specific chromosomal regions, to identify one or all of the centromeres and to detect subtelomeric regions or chromosome bands.

Karyotype analysis is indicated in sexual differentiation disorders and in alterations of spermatogenesis in male infertility. The frequency of chromosomal aberrations in infertile men is 6%, 10 times more frequent than in male newborns. It is recommended to perform a karyotype analysis in the presence of oligozoospermia (sperm count less than 10 million/mL), or in the presence of a family history of multiple abortions, infertility, or chromosomal abnormalities.

Numerical Aberrations

Klinefelter syndrome is the most common numerical chromosomal abnormality, with an incidence in males of 1:500. It is characterized by aneuploidy of the sex chromosomes, which in its most common form consists of a supernumerary X chromosome (XXY). It is the most common cause of non-obstructive azoospermia, with an incidence of 11% in azoospermic men. The karyotype can also show a mosaicism like 46,XY/47,XXY. In these cases the presence of a normal cell line 46, XY can produce a simple oligozoospermia. The identification of the normal cell line is of paramount importance, as it is a marker of the presence of isolated foci of spermatogenesis, and is therefore a positive prognostic factor for assisted reproduction techniques.

Sperm chromosome studies in men with Klinefelter syndrome have demonstrated that the supernumerary X chromosome is eliminated during spermatogenesis. This means that the majority of the children of these men have a normal set of chromosomes, but the risk of chromosomal abnormalities in the fetus is still higher than in the general population.

Men with Klinefelter syndrome present with a phenotype variable from normal to androgen deficiency; the severity of the phenotype appears to correlate with the number of supernumerary X chromosomes. At birth there are no substantial differences with normal newborns, although there seems to be a higher incidence of cryptorchidism. The clinical manifestations appear during puberty, when the increase of gonadotropins is not matched by an increase of the seminiferous tubules, which instead undergo a hyaline degeneration, so that the testes remain small (<5 mL) and hard.

The dysfunction of Leydig cells involves a variable reduction in testosterone production and an increase of LH with a consequent increase in the secretion of estrogen and gynecomastia. The subjects generally are high, due to the delay in fusion of the epiphyseal plates of the long bones, resulting in a eunuchoid habitus. There may be a higher incidence of cryptorchidism, diabetes mellitus, obesity, hypothyroidism, cardiovascular disease, chronic lung diseases such as COPD, varicose veins and venous thromboembolism, breast cancer, and autoimmune diseases. Sometimes children with Klinefelter syndrome have dyslexia, speech problems, learning difficulties and decreased intelligence. Serum levels of testosterone may be decreased or normal, estradiol can be high, and LH and FSH levels may be normal or elevated.

At puberty, the testes develop a fibrohyalinosis of the wall of the tubules, which evolves rapidly in gonadal atrophy by apoptosis of germ cells. However, some cells 47,XXY are able to produce normal sperm, and there can also be individual residual foci of spermatogenesis in azoospermic men. Semen analysis reveals azoospermia or severe oligozoospermia. This leads to the need to cryopreserve semen as soon as possible, before the entire testicle has degenerated.

Another numerical chromosomal aberration is the male with karyotype 46,XX (de la Chapelle syndrome). This disorder affects 1:20,000 men. During paternal meiosis, the aberrant translocation of material to the X chromosome from the Y chromosome, including the region of sex determination (SRY), produces a male with a karyotype 46,XX. The presence of SRY genes leads to the differentiation of the testis, but the absence of the long arm of the Y chromosome leads to the absence of spermatogenesis. These men have a normal sexual development with normal external genitalia, but a higher incidence of hypospadias and cryptorchidism.

The syndrome with karyotype 47,XYY (Jacob's syndrome or chromosome Y disomy) is more common in infertile males, although most men with karyotype 47,XYY have normal offspring. It is believed that this happens because these men lose the supernumerary Y chromosome during spermatogenesis. 47,XYY syndrome occurs in about 1:1,000 newborn males, and is associated with an increased risk of learning disabilities and delayed development of language skills.

Structural Alterations

Structural alterations of the chromosomes include translocations (a large part of a chromosome breaks off and attaches to another chromosome), inversions (a segment of a chromosome is broken, inverted, and reinserted into the chromosome at the same breakage site), insertions (a small segment of a chromosome is inserted into another chromosome), ring chromosomes (aberrant circular chromosomes), *etc.* It is important to identify individuals with translocations or inversions among couples undergoing ICSI, because in case of a pregnancy the likelihood of chromosomal abnormalities in the offspring is increased. Translocations and other hereditary chromosomal disorders can be the cause of a family history of recurrent abortions.

Robertsonian translocations are the most common structural chromosomal rearrangements in infertile men. They result from the fusion of the long arms of two acrocentric chromosomes. Acrocentric chromosomes are chromosomes with one arm much longer than the other, and are the Y chromosome and the chromosomes 13, 14, 15, 21, and 22. The two long arms form an abnormal chromosome, while the short arms are usually lost, so the carrier has 45 chromosomes. The gametes of the Robertsonian translocation carriers can be normal or aneuploid with an extra or missing long arm. The offspring may be affected by Down or Patau syndrome.

Reciprocal translocations occur when there is an exchange of genetic material between homologous chromosomes. Many of these translocations lead to an increase in fetal mortality.

Y Chromosome Abnormalities

The Y chromosome is present only in males and is one of the smallest human chromosomes (60Mb). It is very rich in non-coding sequences, so that for a long time it has been considered inert from a genetic point of view. Now several genes have been identified, which are involved in male sex development. In particular, the region "Male specific Y" (MSY) produces 156 transcripts and contains 27 genes in single and multi-copy. Most of the MSY genes are involved in functions such as male sex determination (SRY) and spermatogenesis. Consequently, deletions or mutations in these genes can lead to defects in spermatogenesis or to "sex reversal". The phenomenon of sex reversal occurs when there is a translocation of SRY on the X chromosome, so that there can be male XX individuals and female XY individuals.

There are three main genetic alterations of the Y chromosome associated with male infertility: AZF microdeletions, partial deletions of the AZFc region (gr/gr) and Y chromosome haplogroups.

The Y chromosome microdeletions affect particular regions of the long arm of the Y chromosome called AZF (AZoospermia Factor). These are fragile regions, because they are made from blocks of repeated multicopy genes with mirror structure, which predisposes to the loss of genetic material. The break points are the same also in different unrelated individuals: there are five break points with five possible types of microdeletions. However, from a clinical point of view, there are only three important types of microdeletions, namely the deletion AZFa, AZFb and AZFc, and the combination AZFb + c. The term "microdeletions" is not totally appropriate because in reality there is a loss of thousands and thousands of bases from the Y chromosome during meiosis, enough to be discovered in 1976 because they are visible under light microscopy.

Deletions of the AZF regions are the most common known genetic cause of severe oligozoospermia and azoospermia, and there is a direct cause-effect relationship between the AZF deletions and abnormalities of spermatogenesis. The frequency in the general population is approximately 1:4,000, in men with severe oligozoospermia is 5–7%, and in men with azoospermia is 10–18%. Microdeletions of the AZF regions have not been found in normozoospermic subjects, indicating that the Y chromosome microdeletions are always associated with damage of spermatogenesis. Typically, these abnormalities are not transmitted to the offspring.

The loss of genetic material may begin during the embryogenesis of the infertile male, but most probably it happened during the spermatogenesis of his father. During a normal spermatogenesis a sperm with the AZFa deletion will appear every 100,000 sperm (the frequency of other microdeletions has not been studied). The child born from this deleted sperm will present the same deletion, with a variable azoospermic, cryptozoospermic or oligozoospermic phenotype.

The AZFa deletion causes the Sertoli Cell Only (SCO) syndrome, and the AZFb deletion causes spermatogenesis arrest at meiosis with an accumulation of primary spermatocytes. In both cases, despite normal testicular volume and normal FSH levels, the spermatozoa do not complete their maturation and are incapable of fertilization even if they are used in ICSI. For this reason the presence of the complete AZFa and AZFb deletion is a contraindication to testicular biopsy to extract sperm (TEsticular Sperm Extraction - TESE). All azoospermic or severe oligozoospermic infertile men need to perform genetic testing before TESE, varicocelectomy, or ICSI. In case of the complete deletion of AZFa and AZFb TESE should not be recommended because the subjects are sterile.

The AZFc region, which contains several genes involved in spermatogenesis, is a highly unstable chromosomal region that may experience recombination events responsible for microdeletions, partial deletions and/or duplications. Microdeletions of this region are the most frequent and the least severe, as in 50% of cases there is the possibility of finding foci of normal spermatogenesis. Aging men with this type of deletion progressively lose the capacity for normal spermatogenesis and their spermiogram worsens until it develops azoospermia. So finding a deletion of the AZFc region in a young man, who still produces normal sperm, is an indication for semen cryopreservation, a simple and inexpensive method that safeguards their childbearing potential in the future. Some of these men also have karyotype abnormalities because they lose the deleted Y chromosome and form a mosaicism 46,XY/45,X0. The presence of mosaicism worsens the spermatogenic function and these men are almost always azoospermic.

The offspring of men with Y chromosome microdeletions has an increased risk of having a karyotype 45,X0 (Turner syndrome), 47,XXY (Klinefelter syndrome), or mosaics due to the loss of the Y chromosome. Microdeletions of the Y chromosome are also often associated with hypogonadotropic hypogonadism, cryptorchidism, and varicocele, so they should be suspected in all cases of azoospermia and oligozoospermia (sperm concentration < 5 million/mL in non-idiopathic forms and < 10 million/mL in idiopathic forms).

Male infertility is also significantly associated with the gr/gr deletion of the AZFc region of the Y chromosome, which increases the risk of oligozoospermia by eight times. This deletion removes about half of all genes in the region, and changes the number of copies (gene dosage) of the genes expressed in the germ line, but not to the same extent of the deletion of the entire AZFc region. Consequently, these deletions are a risk factor for oligo-azoospermia but are also observed in normozoospermic men. As the number of genetic rearrangements increases, so does the reduction of spermatogenic potential, because of the presence of genomic instability. Even the gr/gr deletions are transmitted to the male offspring and thus their identification is important for genetic counselling. There are no associations between paternal deletion of the AZF regions and cryptorchidism or testicular cancer in the male offspring, but the presence of the gr/gr deletion doubles the risk of testicular cancer in the carrier.

Polymorphisms and Mutations

The human genome shows an extraordinary natural variability that manifests itself in various ways, the most frequent of which are the single nucleotide polymorphisms (SNPs, pronounced "snips") consisting of exchanges of individual nucleotides, the variable number of tandem repeats (VNTR), based on changes in the number of repetitive sequences, and the copy number variations (CNV), based on deletions or duplications of DNA sequences which can be long, sometimes as much as several million base pairs.

Polymorphisms are natural variations in a gene, DNA sequence or chromosome that occur with fairly high frequency in the general population (at least 1%). Below that frequency the genome variations are called mutations. Polymorphisms have no adverse effects on the carrier and can be transmitted to the offspring because they not involve major functional changes. Most polymorphisms are located in DNA areas where no gene is involved and therefore are neutral, or they can be near genes that could affect transcription and the amount of the transcript, with advantages or disadvantages or neutral effects. Thus, polymorphisms may be risk factors or protective factors with respect to specific diseases. It is possible that some polymorphisms only lead to dysfunction when associated to a specific genetic background or environmental factor.

Polymorphisms are also present in genes involved in spermatogenesis and in its regulation, and may have a role as risk factors for male infertility. There are significant associations with male infertility for the mutation of the MTHFR (methylenetetrahydrofolate) gene located on chromosome 1. This gene encodes an enzyme that catalyses the conversion of 5,10-methylenetetrahydrofolate to 5-methyltetrahydrofolate, a substrate used to convert the potentially toxic homocysteine to methionine. The mutation 677C→T increases by 39% the incidence of infertility ($p < 0.001$) because it reduces the activity of the enzyme and leads to an alteration of folate metabolism, essential for DNA methylation and for spermatogenesis. The MTHFR polymorphism is a significant risk factor mainly in countries with low folate intake such as India. Another significant association with male infertility is the deletion gr/gr of the AZFc region of the Y chromosome. Other promising polymorphisms in the context of male infertility are that of protamine, associated with teratozoospermia with high DNA fragmentation, and the genes of the endocrine regulation of spermatogenesis, particularly in relation to the exposure to xenoestrogens, underlying the function of the interaction between environment and genetic background.

The androgen receptor (AR) is a nuclear receptor that is activated by the binding of the androgenic hormones testosterone and dihydrotestosterone (DHT). Its main functions are to act as a transcription factor that binds to DNA and regulates gene expression. Its gene is located on the proximal part of the long arm of the X chromosome (locus Xq11-Xq12). It consists of about 2,757 nucleotides divided into eight exons. Like other nuclear receptors, the AR protein has several functional domains: the domain of regulation of transcription, which binds to various transcription factors (exon 1), the DNA binding domain (in exons 2 and 3) and the domain of the link with steroids (from exon 4 to exon 8). More than 400 mutations of the AR had been described by 2010, and the number continues to grow. Inheritance is maternal and typically follows an X-linked recessive model: individuals with a 46,XY karyotype always express the mutated gene because there is only one X chromosome, while carriers of the karyotype 46,XX will not be affected by the mutation because the other X chromosome is not mutated. In 30% of cases, the mutation of AR is spontaneous and not hereditary. Not all mutations in the AR gene are functional, because not all change an amino acid and even when they do they can give rise to different phenotypes of resistance, or insensitivity, to androgens. The phenotypic spectrum of androgen resistance in a carrier of the 46,XY karyotype with a mutation of the AR extends from Morris syndrome (complete androgen insensitivity, CAIS, with female external genitalia at birth) to Reifenstein syndrome (partial androgen insensitivity, PAIS, with ambiguous external genitalia at birth) to the hypovirilized male (mild androgen insensitivity, MAIS, with male external genitalia). The gonads in these individuals are male, since the testicles develop according to an androgen-independent mechanism, but they are often localized in the abdomen. The testosterone produced by the testes is aromatized to estrogens and is therefore responsible for the observed feminization. Spermatogenesis is blocked at an early stage and the subject is usually infertile. The search for AR mutations must not be done routinely in infertile men, because many mutations have not been shown to have a functional role, but should be sought only in selected cases of male infertility, when the man is hypovirilized, has a history of cryptorchidism, and has a high degree of androgen resistance indicated by elevated testosterone and LH levels.

On the androgen receptor gene, in exon 1, there is a polymorphic region of CAG trinucleotide repeats (CAG repeats) that encode a glutamine. The length of this region, which is called the polyglutaminic region, affects the transactivation activity of the AR, because it attracts the amount of transcription factors and changes the final product of transcription. Some studies have shown that if the polyglutaminic region is shorter, androgenicity increases, while if the region is longer, there is less androgenicity, associated with male infertility and less masculinized genitalia in men [7]. The average number of repeats varies according to ethnicity: Caucasians exhibit an average of 21 CAG repeats, while (for example) Africans will exhibit an average of 18 and Chinese 23. Such differences could explain the different degrees of androgenization of various ethnic groups. Several studies have associated the risk of azoospermia and severe oligozoospermia to the expansion of the CAG repeats beyond 26. In men, the number of CAG repeats is also associated with pathological states, for example prostate cancer, hepatocellular carcinoma, and mental retardation are associated with a very low number of repetitions. In women a short polyglutaminic region of the AR has been associated with polycystic ovary syndrome.

A specific mutation of a gene, the cystic fibrosis transmembrane conductance regulator (CFTR) gene, is the cause of cystic fibrosis (CF) and obstructive azoospermia. CF is the most common fatal autosomal recessive disorder in the white population, with an incidence of about 1:2,500 live births. More than 550 mutations have been described for the CFTR gene, with 51 mutations being most common in most ethnic groups. Men with CF have a wide spectrum of disease manifestations, with milder forms characterized by a history of recurrent respiratory infections as a child and teenager, bronchial asthma, and a family history of recurrent respiratory disease or infertility. About 95% men with CF have congenital bilateral absence of the vas deferens (CBAVD), malformations of the epididymis, and atrophy or absence of seminal vesicles and ejaculatory ducts. Testosterone levels are normal and spermatogenesis is usually normal, so men with CF have the ability to generate using Testicular Sperm Aspiration (TESA) and in vitro fertilization.

The role of genetic alterations in diseases of sperm motility is not clear. There are 200 proteins associated to the axoneme of the flagellum of the sperm, but few have been characterized. Dynein is the main protein responsible for flagellar movement. Any alteration of the dynein genes may alter not only the sperm flagellar movement, but also the movement of all ciliated and flagellate cells, resulting in asthenozoospermia and infertility, chronic respiratory disease, and deafness. Kartagener's syndrome is characterized by abnormalities of the dynein genes resulting in complete immobility of spermatozoa, bronchiectasis, chronic sinusitis and situs inversus.

Epigenetics

Genetic causes explain only 15% cases of male infertility, but a new branch of genetics, epigenetics, may be able to better explain the etiology of male infertility. The genome consists of the information encoded by the sequence of nucleotides in DNA, whereas the epigenome consists of all those variations of the structure of DNA and histones that regulate and modify gene expression without changing the sequence of DNA nucleotides. Epigenetic changes (such as DNA methylation, post-translational modifications of histones and chromatin remodelling) may have short or long-term effects and may also be transmitted to the offspring [8]. The epigenetic regulation is strongly influenced by environmental stimuli and endocrine disruptors probably act by this mechanism.

CONCLUSION

Male infertility can be caused by a genetic problem. In general, genetic testing is required when azoospermia or severe oligozoospermia are present, or in case of hypogonadotropic hypogonadism with evident family history. Genetic diagnosis is important for assessing the genetic risk for any offspring and to clarify the diagnosis. The indications for genetic testing are summarized in Appendix 1.

CONSENT FOR PUBLICATION

Not applicable.

CONFLICT OF INTEREST

The author (editor) declares no conflict of interest, financial or otherwise.

ACKNOWLEDGEMENTS

Declared none.

FURTHER READING

Jungwirth A, Giwercman A, Tournaye H, *et al*. European Association of Urology guidelines on male infertility: the 2012 update. Eur Urol 2012; 62(2): 324–32.

Hamada A, Esteves SC, Agarwal A. Unexplained male infertility: potential causes and management. Hum Androl 2011; 1: 2–16.

Krausz C. Male infertility: Pathogenesis and clinical diagnosis. Best Pract Res Clin Endocrinol Metab 2011; 25: 271–85.

Nieschlag E, Behre HM, Nieschlag S. Andrology: Male Reproductive Health and Dysfunction. Heidelberg, Germany: Springer 2010.

Rey RA, Grinspon RP. Normal male sexual differentiation and aetiology of disorders of sex development. Best Pract Res Clin Endocrinol Metab 2011; 25(2): 221–38.

Sharpe RM. Environmental/lifestyle effects on spermatogenesis. Philos Trans R Soc Lond B Biol Sci 2010; 365(1546): 1697–712

BIBLIOGRAPHY

[1]   Skakkebaek NE, Rajpert-De Meyts E, Main KM. Testicular dysgenesis syndrome: an increasingly common developmental disorder with environmental aspects. Hum Reprod 2001; 16(5): 972-8.
[http://dx.doi.org/10.1093/humrep/16.5.972] [PMID: 11331648]

[2]   Sikka SC, Wang R. Endocrine disruptors and estrogenic effects on male reproductive axis. Asian J Androl 2008; 10(1): 134-45.
[http://dx.doi.org/10.1111/j.1745-7262.2008.00370.x] [PMID: 18087652]

[3]   Skinner MK, Manikkam M, Guerrero-Bosagna C. Epigenetic transgenerational actions of endocrine disruptors. Reprod Toxicol 2011; 31(3): 337-43.
[http://dx.doi.org/10.1016/j.reprotox.2010.10.012] [PMID: 21055462]

[4]   Jensen TK, Gottschau M, Madsen JO, *et al.* Habitual alcohol consumption associated with reduced semen quality and changes in reproductive hormones; a cross-sectional study among 1221 young Danish men. BMJ Open 2014; 4(9): e005462.
[http://dx.doi.org/10.1136/bmjopen-2014-005462] [PMID: 25277121]

[5]   Ford WC, North K, Taylor H, Farrow A, Hull MG, Golding J. Increasing paternal age is associated with delayed conception in a large population of fertile couples: evidence for declining fecundity in older men. Hum Reprod 2000; 15(8): 1703-8.
[http://dx.doi.org/10.1093/humrep/15.8.1703] [PMID: 10920089]

[6]   Carrell DT. The genetics of male infertility. New York City, NY: Humana Press 2007.
[http://dx.doi.org/10.1007/978-1-59745-176-5]

[7]   Rajpert-De Meyts E, Leffers H, Petersen JH, *et al.* CAG repeat length in androgen-receptor gene and reproductive variables in fertile and infertile men. Lancet 2002; 359(9300): 44-6.
[http://dx.doi.org/10.1016/S0140-6736(02)07280-X] [PMID: 11809188]

[8]   Rajender S, Avery K, Agarwal A. Epigenetics, spermatogenesis and male infertility. Mutat Res 2011; 727(3): 62-71.
[http://dx.doi.org/10.1016/j.mrrev.2011.04.002] [PMID: 21540125]

CHAPTER 3

Clinical Approach to Male Infertility

Abstract: The clinical approach to the infertile man begins with a careful medical history and physical examination, assessing both the andrological and internal medicine aspects. The main objectives of the evaluation are to identify modifiable risk factors and appropriate treatments which may improve male fertility, and to exclude the presence of comorbidities such as testicular cancer, osteoporosis, and endocrine or genetic problems that can be associated with infertility. The laboratory tests described include the evaluation of endocrine tests, of the spermiogram and of genetic studies.

Keywords: Antisperm Aantibody, Asthenozoospermia, Azoospermia, DNA Fragmentation, Fluidification, FSH, LH, Karyotype, Medical History, Micro-deletions of the Y Chromosome, Nonprogressive Motility, Oligozoospermia, Progressive motility, Pulsatile Prolactin, SHBG, Spermiogram, Teratozoospermia, Testicular Biopsy, Testicular Fine Needle Aspiration, Viscosity.

CLINICAL HISTORY

The clinical approach to the infertile man begins with a careful medical history and physical examination, assessing both the andrological and internal medicine aspects. The main objectives of the evaluation are to identify modifiable risk factors and appropriate treatments which may improve male fertility, and to exclude the presence of comorbidities such as testicular cancer, osteoporosis, and endocrine or genetic problems that can be associated with infertility.

The main areas of investigation are the following:

General Information: age, race, profession, primary or secondary infertility, duration of infertility.

Family History: family history of infertility, miscarriages, multiple abortions, stillbirths, genetic diseases and endocrine diseases, recurrent congenital malformations.

Occupational History and Lifestyle: environmental factors and occupational exposure, eating habits, sports, alcohol, smoking, drug use, sauna, tight pants, long-term use of bicycle riding and horse riding.

Sexual History: frequency of sexual intercourse, libido, erection, ejaculation characteristics, characteristics of orgasm, use of lubricants, hematospermia, anejaculation, presence or history of sexually transmitted diseases, difficulty with bowel movements; if there are problems with ejaculation, investigate the turbidity of urine after ejaculation and if there is a decrease in volume of ejaculate.

Past Medical History: mumps after 11 years of age, chronic diseases of the upper respiratory tract, chronic sinusitis, bronchiectasis, COPD, cystic fibrosis, tuberculosis, chronic infections, cancer, chemotherapy and/or radiotherapy, allergies, thyroid disease, hyperprolactinemia, diabetes mellitus, adrenal diseases, renal and hepatic failure, hemochromatosis, neurological diseases, and fever that occurred in the previous three months.

Use of Drugs: in particular antibiotics, calcium channel blockers, spironolactone, and other anabolic androgens, over the counter drugs.

Diseases of the Urogenital System: cryptorchidism, precocious or delayed puberty, testicular trauma and/or torsion, orchitis, sexually transmitted diseases, epididymitis, prostatitis, vesiculitis, urethritis, genital dermatoses.

Surgery of the Genital Tract: history of orchidopexy, orchiectomy, interventions for inguinal hernia, detorsion of the spermatic cord, varicocelectomy, hydrocelectomy, epididimovasostomy, prostatectomy, bladder interventions, surgery for hypospadias, circumcision.

History of the Female Partner: any previous pregnancies (including miscarriages or elective terminations), length of menstrual cycle, if she is being evaluated for fertility problems, any medical or surgical treatment for fertility.

Other: anosmia, peripheral visual field defects, pain or fluids leaking from the breast, scrotal pain, weight gain or loss, sleep apnea syndrome, situs inversus.

GENERAL PHYSICAL EXAMINATION

Measurement of vital signs: blood pressure; weight and height to calculate the Body Mass Index (BMI, weight in kilograms divided by the square of height in meters); waist circumference. General physical examination and review of secondary sexual characteristics (hair thinning and female distribution may be a sign of hypo-androgenism). A possible gynecomastia can result from exposure to endogenous or exogenous estrogens, or drugs such as spironolactone or digitalis.

UROGENITAL PHYSICAL EXAMINATION

The exam covers:

Penis: the inspection should identify possible presence of hypospadias, phimosis or short frenulum, trauma or surgery scars, fibrotic plaques, inflammatory lesions.

Testicles: the examination must be carried out with the man standing in a warm room (24–25°C), the testes must be present in the scrotum and palpable, with a hard-elastic consistency and without nodules.

Epididymis: light palpation to exclude the presence of tenderness or nodules.

Vas Deferens: must be palpable and mobile.

Testicular Volumes: measured with orchidometer.

Varicoceles: possibly detectable with the Valsalva maneuver.

Inguinal Examination: to identify any surgical scars, signs of infection and enlarged lymph nodes.

Rectal Examination: to examine the accessory glands and the prostate.

LABORATORY TESTS

The most important tests include:

• Sperm analysis or spermiogram (see below); if the result is abnormal in two properly collected specimens, the semen analysis should be repeated after 4–6 weeks.

• Colour Doppler ultrasonography: examination of the testis (size, shape, location and echogenicity), epididymis and didymus; arterial and venous flow parameters.

• Dosage of FSH, LH and testosterone (only in patients with azoospermia or severe oligo-astheno-teratozoospermia and signs of hypogonadism) to differentiate the origin of hypogonadism of testicular origin (primary or hypergonadotropic) from that of central origin (or secondary hypogonadism) (see Table **10**). The value of FSH is inversely related to the spermatogenic function: if FSH is high, it is indicative of primitive testicular damage, if FSH is normal, it is indicative of an obstructive form, or primitive testicular damage, if FSH is low and associated with azoospermia it is indicative of hypogonadotropic hypogonadism. The value of LH is related to the steroidogenic function: if LH is high it indicates severe testicular damage or androgen insensitivity, if LH is low and associated with low levels of FSH it is indicative of central hypogonadism.

Other tests, which should be performed in selected cases, include:

• Blood glucose, urethral swab: to be measured in the presence of urinary frequency, dysuria, and tenderness of the epididymis, or if the semen analysis shows asthenozoospermia, pH > 8, high viscosity and/or leukocytospermia.

Table 10. Hormonal values in various forms of male infertility.

Causes	LH	FSH	Testosterone
Pre-testicular	↓	↓	↓
Pre-testicular (exogenous androgens)	↓	↓	↑
Testicular	↑	↑	↓
Testicular (androgen insensibility)	↑	↑	↑
Post-testicular	Normal	Normal	Normal

Legend: ↑ = above normal value; ↓ = below normal value.

GENETIC STUDIES (IN THE PRE-TESTICULAR, TESTICULAR AND POST-TESTICULAR FORMS)

1. Karyotype, in case of a family history of infertility and recurrent pregnancy loss, primary testicular failure and small testes and in all subjects with less than 10 million sperm/mL.

2. Molecular studies:

• Mutations in the CFTR gene, in case of subjects with obstructive azoospermia and bilateral agenesis of the vas deferens, or with oligozoospermia and unilateral absence of the vas deferens.

• Microdeletions of the Y chromosome, in case of subjects with less than 5 million sperm/mL, if infertility is associated with varicocele, cryptorchidism, hypogonadotropic hypogonadism or obstructive forms, or with idiopathic infertility and less than 10 million sperm/mL.

• Mutations in the androgen receptor in the case of subjects with elevated FSH and testosterone.

TESTICULAR SPERM RETRIEVAL

Testicular sperm retrieval is a necessary procedure to evaluate spermatogenesis in patients with azoospermia, in order to differentiate obstructive *vs* non-obstructive azoospermia. It can be done by percutaneous testicular fine needle aspiration (TEFNA) or by open testicular biopsy (TESE).

A significant proportion of men with azoospermia, normal testicular size and normal FSH levels in reality may have severe spermatogenetic disorders, such as hypospermatogenesis (presence of all cellular elements of spermatogenesis but reduced in number), arrest of spermatogenesis (presence of cellular elements of spermatogenesis only up to a certain stage), and the Only Sertoli cell syndrome or germ cell aplasia (the tubules contain Sertoli cells but not germ cells). However in many cases there may be foci of active spermatogenesis, which would make it possible to perform ICSI. In these cases of non-obstructive azoospermia testicular biopsy (TESE) provides an adequate amount of cells for cytologic diagnosis and possibly for ICSI. In obstructive azoospermia, spermatogenesis is normal, and testicular biopsy helps recover sperm upstream from the occlusion, for later use in ICSI.

TESE damages the testis, particularly if multiple withdrawals are made at various points of the testis, because it increases the likelihood of damaging the branches of the testicular artery. These phenomena of devascularization sometimes become permanent and can be associated with a transient decrease in testosterone levels, which returns to normal within about 18 months. For this reason, the best approach in azoospermic men is to schedule a diagnostic TESE and simultaneously to cryopreserve the removed tissue for one or more subsequent ICSI. This is to avoid multiple sampling at each cycle of IVF, resulting in damage to the remaining testicle, and to avoid the risk of not having recovered some sperm on the day of fertilization after stimulating the female partner.

If patients with non-obstructive azoospermia are candidates for ICSI, before performing TESE they should be investigated for microdeletions of the Y chromosome, because the complete deletion of the region AZFa or AZFb or AZFb + c deletions of regions make a man sterile, so it is useless to seek sperm for fertilization.

SPERMIOGRAM

Every male partner of an infertile couple should undergo a semen analysis. Semen analysis is a diagnostic test performed on the seminal fluid, to assess the amount and concentration of spermatozoa, their motility and morphology, the presence of anti-sperm antibodies and the percentage of live sperm. Despite being an examination of fundamental importance in the diagnostic workup of the infertile couple, it does not give any direct information on the fertility of the subject. It cannot unambiguously discriminate between the fertile and infertile male, except in cases of azoospermia or necrozoospermia, and its results usually present great variability, so it should always be repeated at least once after 4–6 weeks. Given the complexity of semen analysis each seminology laboratory should use specialized personnel and quality instruments, and utilize a program of both internal and external quality control.

The World Health Organization (WHO) periodically publishes the "WHO laboratory manual for the examination of seminal fluid", which lists all the procedures for the proper performance of semen analysis [1]. The new 2010 edition of the Manual provides new thresholds of normality for various seminal parameters which in several cases are much lower than in previous editions. These changes were motivated by new scientific evidence based on large numbers of men of proven fertility. The values chosen as lower reference values are based on the 5ᵗʰ percentile of the distribution of the data; this means that 5% of men with those values are certainly fertile, but this certainly is a very low rate of fertility! Actually, there is considerable overlap in the various parameters of the semen analysis among infertile and fertile men, so that no measure is truly diagnostic of infertility. Table **11** lists the values of the main semen parameters of fertile men according to the latest edition of the WHO Manual.

Table 11. Distribution of the values of semen parameters of fertile men according to the WHO Manual (2010).

Seminal parameters	5ᵗʰ percentile	50ᵗʰ percentile
Seminal volume (mL)	1.5	3.7
Concentration (10^6/mL)	15	73
Total number (10^6/ejaculate)	39	255
Total motility (PR+NP, %)	40	61
Progressive motility (PR, %)	32	55
Normal forms (%)	4	15
Vitality (%)	58	79

Legend: PR: progressive motility; NP: non-progressive motility; 5ᵗʰ percentile = threshold of the seminal parameter value below which less than 5% men conceived a child; 50ᵗʰ percentile = threshold of the seminal parameter value below which less than 50% men conceived a child.

PRE-ANALYTICAL FACTORS

The semen collection should be done exclusively by masturbation after a minimum of 2–3 days and a maximum of 5–7 days of sexual abstinence. Abstinence can affect sperm concentration, but it does not affect motility or vitality. The freshly collected sample must be maintained at 37°C and examined one hour after ejaculation, and no later than two hours. The man should report any loss of seminal fluid, and if the loss is at the beginning or at the end of the emission, because the first part of the ejaculate is richer in spermatozoa and its loss leads to a significant alteration of sperm concentration. The collection should occur at the laboratory of seminology, although it may be permitted at home provided that the sample is maintained at 37°C and is delivered to the laboratory within one hour. The container must be sterile.

Other factors that may affect the quality of semen analysis are the presence of a high fever, or taking antibiotics, in the two months prior to the exam. In this case it is better to postpone the execution of the examination.

Macroscopic Evaluation

The volume of the ejaculate is considered normal if it is > 1.5 mL, with physiological changes in relation to the duration of abstinence. It comes mostly (90%) from the accessory glands. In the case of an obstructive or inflammatory dysfunction of these glands the volume of the seminal fluid is reduced. The volume also depends on the level of androgenization, because testosterone is important for prostate and seminal vesicles health. In case of hypoandrogenization (low testosterone levels), there is a lower production of seminal fluid because the prostate and seminal vesicles are less developed. The absence of seminal fluid with orgasm is called aspermia.

The seminal fluid normally is opalescent and homogeneous; in case of azoospermia or severe oligozoospermia it may have a transparent watery appearance. A milky colour, especially if it is accompanied by azoospermia, may indicate an ejaculate consisting largely of prostatic secretion. A yellowish colour is indicative of the presence of a significant number of white blood cells (piospermia), while a pinkish or darker colour is indicative of the presence of red blood cells (hemospermia).

The viscosity of the seminal fluid is about six times greater than that of water. It is a rheological characteristic common to all bodily fluids and depends on their biochemical and cytological composition. A modification of the viscosity is indicative of a pathology of the accessory glands or of a local inflammation, or it may be due to a systemic disease of the exocrine secretions.

The fluidification is evaluated by percolating semen from a pipette on the walls of a tube and observing the fluid in transparency against a light source. The process of fluidification occurs in a time range between 10 and 60 minutes. After two hours, in the presence of clots or filaments, it is considered incomplete.

The semen pH is generally between 7.2 to 7.8; slightly alkaline values allow the survival of spermatozoa in the vaginal area before the penetration of the cervical mucus.

Sperm Concentration

In fertile men (age range 20–40 years), who are normal from an anatomical, uro-andrological and endocrinological point of view, there is considerable fluctuation in the number of sperm, even in the ejaculates of the same individual.

The number of spermatozoa should be calculated both per mL (concentration) and per total ejaculate (absolute number). The minimum concentration is set at 15 million/mL, while the amount per ejaculate should be at least 39 million/mL.

In case of absence of sperm, to make a differential diagnosis between cryptozoospermia (spermatozoa present but in very small amounts) and azoospermia (no sperm in the ejaculate), every time the ejaculate must be cytocentrifuged to search for sperm in the sediment. If azoospermia is associated with lower than normal volume and pH, an obstruction of the seminal tract may be suspected.

Sperm Motility

Normal sperm advance with a progressive motion according to the direction of its major axis, generated by the beat of the tail. The acquisition of the kinetic properties is a relatively late event in the ontogenetic process of the gamete. In fact, the sperm in the rete testis are immobile; they acquire the ability to move in the epididymis.

Sperm motility is assessed either subjectively by direct observation under an optical microscope, or with various objective computerized techniques. Sperm motility is classified as progressive (PR), nonprogressive (NP), and immotile. The lower reference value for progressive motility is 32%, while for total motility (PR + NP) it is 40%.

Sperm Morphology

The percentage of sperm with normal morphology is the parameter of the spermiogram in vitro which best correlates with the fertilizing capacity of that seminal fluid. The morphology of the sperm is evaluated in every cellular district (head, neck and tail). The lower reference value for morphology is 4%.

Sperm Vitality

Vitality (or viability) is evaluated when the progressive motility is less than 40%, because it is important to know how many immotile sperm are alive or dead. The presence of many immotile but live cells suggests structural defects of the tail, while a high percentage of immotile and non-viable cells may indicate a pathology of the epididymis.

Non-sperm Cells in Semen

Other cellular components can be identified in the seminal fluid. Leukocytes (neutrophils, macrophages and lymphocytes) may suggest the presence of inflammation of the genital tract if more than one million/mL. Red blood cells should not be present in the ejaculate, their presence suggests microhaemorrhages or inflammation. Elements of the germ line are always present, and are usually spermatocytes and spermatids, more rarely spermatogonia.

Epithelial cells, if abundant, indicate inflammation. The prostatic corpuscles are almost never associated with specific prostate disease. The areas of sperm agglutination suggest an autoimmune anti-sperm reaction.

Presence of Anti-sperm Antibodies

The immunological infertility evaluation is based solely on laboratory diagnosis. To demonstrate the presence of antisperm antibody tests use indirect (agglutination) or direct methods (MAR test, antiglobulin Mixed Reaction Test).

To establish a diagnosis of antisperm autoimmunity, however, the mere presence of antisperm antibodies is not sufficient, but it must be demonstrated that the antibodies significantly interfere with sperm function. This can be investigated with a mucus penetration test.

Seminal Plasma Analysis

Some molecules present in the seminal plasma may help in characterizing the obstructive forms. The most useful ones are fructose (secreted by the seminal vesicles), acid phosphatase and zinc (secreted by the prostate) and L-carnitine (by the epididymis). These molecules are low in obstructive cases.

Post-analytical Stage

The report of the seminal examination should include a description of all parameters examined. "Fertility rates" should not be specified, as they are in the best of cases without clinical significance, and often prove misleading.

Sperm Function Testing

The spermiogram provides an initial evaluation of the infertile male, but it is not a test of male fertility. Sperm function testing is used to assess if the sperm have the biological ability to fertilize ova, and to select sperm with the best characteristics for fertilization. It is indicated in case of sperm abnormalities in the spermiogram or if there is "unexplained" couple infertility. The advent of ICSI has decreased the demand for these tests because none of them are predictive of success or failure of ICSI and many couples choose to undergo the treatment anyway, regardless of their result. A variety of tests are available to evaluate different aspects of sperm function, and are summarized in Table **12**.

Table 12. Main sperm function tests.

Test	Function
Swelling test	To evaluate membrane integrity and vitality of sperm
Post coital test	To evaluate the sperm-cervical mucus interaction
Capacitation: swim up test	In normozoospermic males
Capacitation: poor sperm test	In oligo- or asthenozoospermic males
Acrosomal reaction	To evaluate capacitation
Sperm-zona pellucida binding test	Interaction between spermatozoa and zona pellucida
HOPT (Hamster Penetration Ovum Test)	Penetration of spermatozoa in ova

DNA FRAGMENTATION

The spermiogram has a low predictive value for male fertility. In fact, 15–25% infertile males have normozoospermia, while in a population of proven fertile males, who had a conception within one year from the date of the test, only 12% have normozoospermia and the rest have at least one abnormal parameter. On the other hand, sperm DNA fragmentation is present also in a small percentage of spermatozoa from fertile men, but the spermatozoa of infertile men present more DNA damage which negatively affects their fertilizing potential. There is evidence that, for spontaneous pregnancies, increasing DNA fragmentation is related to an increased amount of time required to attain pregnancy, and also to decreased probability of pregnancy. In the case of assisted fertilization, the increase of sperm DNA fragmentation, in particular to levels over 30%, significantly decreases the likelihood of pregnancy.

The DNA of the Y chromosome in the male gametes has a greater likelihood of being damaged. Since there is only one Y chromosome available during meiosis, during recombination there is no repair. For this reason there are several defence measures, for example the sperm DNA is much more compact than the DNA of somatic cells, so the volume of sperm is reduced during the journey through the genital tract, the damage caused by exogenous agents can be minimized and the genome is maintained transcriptionally inactive. In addition to these measures, the spermatozoa are immersed in fluids containing high levels of antioxidants.

Nevertheless, DNA is damaged both during sperm development and in mature sperm.

The presence of a high percentage of sperm with damaged DNA may be a cause of infertility or of repeated miscarriages. The oocyte is able to partially repair the damage in the spermatozoon, but the performance of the repair depends on the type of sperm DNA damage. However in some types of damage, for example the double-stranded cut, during repair a large number of mutations are introduced, which is not compatible with the viability of the zygote.

The conditions associated with high DNA fragmentation include varicocele, advanced paternal age, alcohol abuse, smoking, hypercholesterolemia, elevated BMI and exposure to ionizing radiation, pesticides, organic solvents, heat, heavy metals and alkylating agents. With regard to cancer patients, not only does chemotherapy treatment increases the fragmentation of DNA, but this may also be present before the treatment from the mere presence of the tumour. Studies have shown that in some patients with testicular cancer, and in many patients with Hodgkin lymphoma there are levels of DNA fragmentation of 30% or more, which reduces the fertilizing power of the sperm. In these cases, the decision to cryopreserve a seed so damaged must be evaluated carefully.

The causes of DNA fragmentation are not fully known, and the hypothesized mechanisms include a combination of defects in apoptosis and in chromatin maturation and oxidative stress.

DNA fragmentation can be measured by various techniques based on flow cytometry. With these techniques large numbers of cells can be observed, so the results are statistically more robust and more objective. In particular, the Sperm Chromatin Sensitivity Assay (SCSA) is a flow cytometric technique with standardized protocols whose results are expressed as a percentage of fragmented cells. In this case, the damage shown is the susceptibility of chromatin to denaturation induced from the outside, which does not correspond exactly to DNA fragmentation. The TUNEL test (Terminal deoxynucleotidyl transferase dUTP Nick End Labeling) is a technique that determines true DNA fragmentation. The test Comet is the most sensitive technique, as it measures the fragments of intact sperm DNA that separate in an electrophoretic field like a comet tail (from which the name Comet).

The role of tests for the determination of DNA fragmentation in ART is controversial. They can be recommended in the case of a lack of fertilization of the ovum and in the presence of varicocele.

CONSENT FOR PUBLICATION

Not applicable.

CONFLICT OF INTEREST

The author (editor) declares no conflict of interest, financial or otherwise.

ACKNOWLEDGEMENT

Declared none.

FURTHER READING

Kamel RM. Management of the infertile couple: an evidence-based protocol. Reprod Biol Endocrinol 2010; 8: 21.

Lotti F, Corona G, Krausz C, *et al*. The Infertile Male—3: Endocrinological Evaluation. In: Scrotal Pathology. Bertolotto M, Trombetta C, Eds. Springer-Verlag, 2011; pp. 223–40.

BIBLIOGRAPHY

[1]   WHO Laboratory Manual for the Examination and Processing of Human Semen 5th., 2010. Available from: http://apps.who.int/iris/bitstream/10665/44261/1/9789241547789_eng.pdf?ua=1

CHAPTER 4

Treatment of Male Infertility

Abstract: The medical treatment of male infertility is possible when there is a specific etiological factor that is potentially susceptible to medical care. Hormonal replacement therapy is indicated in hypogonadism with different options depending on the purpose of the treatment. To induce or maintain androgenisation, testosterone should be used, while to induce or maintain spermatogenesis, gonadotropins or GnRH should be used. Hyperprolactinemia can be treated with dopamine agonists. Antibiotic therapy is indicated for symptomatic infections of the genital tract. In idiopathic forms, various empirical treatments have been tried with limited success. Surgical therapy is indicated for congenital or acquired obstruction of the seminal ducts, to extract sperm or testicular tissue, and in varicocele. Assisted reproductive technology, in particular Intracytoplasmic Sperm Injection (ICSI), has revolutionized the prognosis of male infertility, because it has allowed azoospermic men to procreate.

Keywords: Androgens, Antioxidant, Coenzyme Q10, Cryopreservation, Expectant Management, ICSI, Intracytoplasmic Sperm Injection, Intrauterine Insemination, In Vitro Fertilization, IUI, IVF, L-Carnitine, Replacement Therapy, Selenium, Testicular Biopsy, Testosterone, Varicocele, Vitamin C, Vitamin E, Zinc.

PREVENTIVE TREATMENT OF MALE INFERTILITY

There are conditions which are known to develop into infertility, like Klinefelter syndrome, hormonal therapy, chemotherapy, radiotherapy or surgery in the pelvic area, *etc.* In these cases semen cryopreservation will protect the fertility assets. Cryopreservation of semen is a procedure to keep the sperm frozen and reused in a subsequent period. The freezing occurs at a controlled speed, with a process known as vitrification. The vitrification process allows sperm to have higher survival and motility after thawing. Whilst cryopreservation seems to cause damage to the plasma membrane and to the acrosome of sperm and spermatids, so far the results of the literature on ICSI from TESE do not show any statistically significant differences between fresh tissue compared to the cryopreserved one.

In the case of cryptorchidism prevention of infertility depends on the corrective surgery within the first two years of life. In this way the undescended testicle is not exposed to the higher intra-abdominal temperatures, which damage the germinal epithelium.

EXPECTANT MANAGEMENT

Before starting a medical or surgical treatment for infertility, if the woman is fertile and the man has idiopathic infertility, it is possible to suggest a period of *expectant management* to increase the possibility of cumulative conception. It has been calculated that, if the woman is less than 40 years of age, and the couple has regular unprotected sexual intercourse, in the first year the couple's infertility is around 20%, while in the second year the rate is halved. Continuing to try, 25–35% of "infertile" couples will finally have a child without any treatment. The success rates are higher if the couple is young and if infertility is of short duration (< 2 years). If the woman is more than 35 years of age, or if infertility has lasted for more than three years, it is better to use the techniques of assisted reproduction sooner.

The expectant management is useful because it is a low-cost intervention. It is not a passive waiting, but a period of 1–2 years in which lifestyle changes are implemented to promote fertility. In expectant management it is possible to conceive, following specific recommendations. The couple must understand that attempts should be made over more years, having sexual intercourse at least 2–3 times a week (not concentrated on the weekend). The men who suffer from infertility are recommended to eliminate all possible environmental toxins, such as smoking and taking drugs, and to consume no more than 3–4 units of alcohol per day. Coffee and tea do not seem to affect male fertility. Men should also avoid hot baths and hot tubs, because high temperatures slow down the production of sperm. The assumption of exogenous testosterone or androgens such as DHEA (to "improve" sport activities) must be absolutely discouraged because it can impair fertility.

MEDICAL TREATMENT OF MALE INFERTILITY

The medical treatment of male infertility is possible when there is a specific etiological factor that is potentially susceptible to medical care.

In hypogonadism there are different options for replacement therapies depending on the purpose of the treatment. To induce or maintain androgenisation, testosterone should be used, to induce or maintain spermatogenesis, gonadotropins or GnRH should be used. In the latter case, the only candidates for replacement therapy are males with hypogonadotropic or secondary hypogonadism, because in the primitive forms the endogenous gonadotropins are already high or the testicular damage is such that it does not allow the recovery of spermatogenesis. Treatment with gonadotropin (hCG, hMG, purified or recombinant FSH) should be continued for at least 18–24 months before a benefit at the level of spermatogenesis can be seen.

Hyperprolactinemia can be treated with dopamine agonists.

If there are symptomatic infections of the genital tract, antibiotic therapy can lead to the resolution of the infection, but it does not always restore fertility. If the man is asymptomatic and presents a spermiogram with high viscosity, leukocytes, altered pH but negative culture tests, there may be a subclinical infection, whose treatment is not always effective and is a controversial choice. The antibiotic in fact has a negative effect on spermatogenesis so, if the couple is trying to obtain a pregnancy, it is better to wait for 1–2 months before performing a new semen analysis.

The nonsteroidal anti-inflammatory drugs (NSAIDs) are used in case of inflammatory diseases of the male accessory sex glands, such as prostatitis, epididymitis and vesiculitis.

In the presence of antisperm antibodies (ASA), the use of condoms reduces the exposure of the female genital tract to sperm and thus reduces the formation of ASA in cervical mucus. Immunosuppressive therapy with steroids seems to be effective only for low titers of ASA. Sperm washing has yielded conflicting results, and ICSI remains the treatment of choice.

If there are sexual problems such as erectile dysfunction or premature ejaculation, a specific drug therapy or sexological counselling can help improve fertility.

In idiopathic forms, various empirical treatments have been examined, but their effectiveness is controversial because of the lack of large randomized trials. However recent systematic reviews have concluded that some empirical treatments increase the live birth rate [1].

Hormonal treatment with exogenous androgens has been proven ineffective. In the long run exogenous androgens block the production of endogenous testosterone, causing testicular atrophy and azoospermia. Their lack of efficacy was also confirmed by a meta-analysis of more than 1,000 infertile men [2]. Hormonal treatment with anti-estrogens such as clomiphene or tamoxifen, and aromatase inhibitors such as testolactone and anastrozole, were also proven ineffective. The rationale of their use is based on the fact that estrogens derived from the aromatization of testosterone can modulate the secretion of GnRH. On the other hand, hormonal treatment with recombinant FSH in idiopathic infertility with normal levels of FSH had a positive effect on sperm production

Treatment with antioxidants is rational when chronic inflammation is present. However, it is difficult to prove that antioxidants administered from the outside will accumulate within the epididymis. Few studies have tried to measure the concentration of various substances in semen and whether this is sufficient to provide an antioxidant effect. The results of studies using vitamin C, coenzyme Q10, pentoxifylline, selenium and zinc are controversial and inconclusive. Some antioxidant treatments gave consistently positive results and are listed in Table **13** [1]. Note that therapies with L-carnitine alone, or combined with acetyl L-carnitine and Vitamin E have not only improved the spermiogram but also significantly increased the number of live births compared to the untreated group. The conclusions of the position statement from the Italian Society of Andrology and Sexual Medicine (SIAMS) are that "evidence supporting the use of antioxidants for the treatment of male infertility is of low quality", and it is suggested that antioxidants should be administered as empirical treatment in men with idiopathic infertility after a thorough diagnostic workup in the presence of abnormal sperm parameters and an altered sperm DNA fragmentation. The suggested cut-off for pathological values of the sperm DNA fragmentation, given the different methods used to evaluate it and the lack of agreement, is above 20%.

Table 13. Antioxidants substances with a beneficial effect in male infertility.

Substance	Action on the male reproductive system
Vitamin E **(300 mg qd for 6 months)**	Improvement of sperm motility, reduction of lipid peroxidation and improvement of pregnancy rates in men with asthenozoospermia
Glutathione (GSH) **(600 mg qod for 2 months)**	Improvement of sperm motility and morphology in men with varicocele or accessory gland infection
L-carnitine	(3 g qd for 4 months) Improvement of sperm concentration, motility and morphology in men with asthenozoospermia
	(2 g qd for 6 months) Improvement of sperm concentration and motility in men with oligo-astheno-teratozoospermia
L-carnitine (2 g qd) + Acetyl-L-carnitine (1 g qd)	Improvement of sperm motility and vitality in men with prostatitis, vesiculitis and epididymitis

SURGICAL TREATMENT OF MALE INFERTILITY

Surgical therapy is indicated for congenital or acquired obstruction of the seminal ducts, to extract sperm or testicular tissue, and in varicocele. Before performing surgery in the male, it is necessary to evaluate the female partner for the presence of female infertility factors.

In obstructive azoospermia, surgical correction can be made if the obstruction is at the level of the epididymis or in the ductal system. The appearance of sperm can take up to 18 months after recanalization, but on average it takes six months to get motile sperm. Adverse prognostic factors are represented by poor spermatogenesis, absence of sperm in the epididymal fluid, and the concomitant presence of ultrasound abnormalities in the prostate, seminal vesicles and ejaculatory ducts. Despite the technological improvements made by ICSI, microsurgical recanalization remains the most reliable and ethical treatment in the management of obstructive epididymal azoospermia, in terms of the number of term pregnancies and of costs. When planning a surgical recanalization care should be taken to cryopreserve sperm for possible ART.

Sperm retrieval for ART is the second therapeutic option in obstructive azoospermia. Sperm retrieval can be performed from the didymus (in obstructive and non-obstructive azoospermia) or at various levels of the seminal ducts (in obstructive azoospermia, according to the level of obstruction) even though the testis is currently the most widely used recovery site. Table **14** lists the surgical procedures used depending on the level of obstruction.

Table 14. Surgery procedures used depending on the level of obstruction.

Testicular level	TESA (Testicular Sperm Aspiration)
	TESE (Testicular Sperm Extraction)
Epididymal level	PESA (Percutaneous Epidydimal Sperm Aspiration)
	MESA (Microsurgical Epidydimal Sperm Aspiration)
Vas deferens level	MSVA (MicroSurgical Vas Aspiration)
Ejaculatory duct level	STW (Seminal Tract Washout)
	TRUSCA (Transrectal Ultrasonically-guided Sperm Cyst Aspiration)

In case of varicocele, the presence of central hypogonadism must be excluded and genetic studies must be done before surgery. If there is an abnormality of the karyotype and varicocele is not symptomatic, there are no indications for surgery. A meta-analysis of a total of 607 patients with varicocele, after excluding hormonal and karyotype alterations and Y chromosome microdeletions, concluded that there is no evidence that treatment of varicocele in couples with idiopathic infertility improves chances of conception [1].

ASSISTED REPRODUCTIVE TECHNOLOGY

Assisted reproductive technology (ART) refers to any technique that intervenes with the gametes (oocytes and spermatozoa) in order to induce a pregnancy in an infertile couple.

If the woman does not present alterations of the pelvic organs and the man has motile sperm, ART treatment is aimed at increasing the probability of encounter for the oocyte and the sperm. Intrauterine insemination (IUI) is the least expensive method and it is easily repeatable.

If the woman presents with tubal obstruction or if there is severe asthenozoospermia, other more complex techniques of fertilization are needed.

In Vitro Fertilization (IVF) involves the fertilization of the gametes outside the female body. The woman undergoes ovarian stimulation with variable protocols and a tight control of the hormonal changes, of the number of follicles in evolution, and of their progression toward maturity. When it is time the oocytes are collected for IVF, and at the same time the man must provide the seminal fluid. In some cases, a previously frozen semen sample is thawed in order to ensure the successful completion of this phase of the procedure. The oocytes are fertilized in vitro and after 2–3 days pre-embryos are transferred into the uterus through a thin catheter.

The Gamete Intra-Fallopian Transfer (GIFT) is a technique alternative to the IVF particularly suitable in those cases in which the sterility is not related to tubal problems, in cases of idiopathic infertility and in cases of male subfertility. In GIFT, oocytes and sperm are transferred simultaneously in the fallopian tubes, so that fertilization occurs *in vivo*.

The Intracytoplasmic Sperm Injection (ICSI) is a technique that involves the injection of a single sperm directly into the oocyte cytoplasm. The ICSI has revolutionized the prognosis of male infertility, because it has allowed azoospermic men to procreate. While IVF requires at least 1 million viable sperm, ICSI needs just a single sperm. Viable embryos able to give rise to pregnancies can be obtained using sperm taken directly from the epididymis (MESA), from the testis by fine-needle aspiration (TESA) or by testicular biopsy (TESE), or from the precursor cells of the spermatogenetic line (spermatids) isolated also from the ejaculate of these subjects.

There are other lesser-used techniques, including ZIFT (Zygote intrafallopian transfer) and TET (Tubal Embryo Transfer). These techniques involve steps similar to IVF, but they transfer zygotes (ZIFT) or pre-embryos (TET) into the tubes.

CONSENT FOR PUBLICATION

Not applicable.

CONFLICT OF INTEREST

The author (editor) declares no conflict of interest, financial or otherwise.

ACKNOWLEDGEMENT

Declared none.

FURTHER READING

Attia AM, Abou-Setta AM, Al-Inany HG. Gonadotrophins for idiopathic male factor subfertility. Cochrane Database of Systematic Reviews 2013; 8: CD005071.

Bieniek JM, Drabovich AP, Lo KC. Seminal Biomarkers for the evaluation of male infertility. Asian J Androl 2016; 18(3): 426–33.

Jung JH, Seo JT. Empirical medical therapy in idiopathic male infertility: Promise or panacea? Clin Exper Reprod Med 2014; 41(3): 108–14.

McLachlan RI, Krausz C. Clinical evaluation of the infertile male: new options, new challenges. Asian J Androl 2012; 14(1): 3–5.

Showell MG . Antioxidants for male subfertility (Review). The Cochrane Collaboration 2012.

Tiseo BC, Esteves SC, Cocuzza MS. Summary evidence on the effects of varicocele treatment to improve natural fertility in subfertile men. Asian J Androl 2016; 18(2): 239–45.

Will MA, Swain J, Fode M, . The great debate: varicocele treatment and impact on fertility. Fertil Steril 2011; 95: 841–52.

BIBLIOGRAPHY

[1]   Baazeem A, Belzile E, Ciampi A, *et al.* Varicocele and male factor infertility treatment: a new meta-analysis and review of the role of varicocele repair. Eur Urol 2011; 60(4): 796-808.
        [http://dx.doi.org/10.1016/j.eururo.2011.06.018] [PMID: 21733620]

[2]   Calogero AE, Aversa A, La Vignera S, Corona G, Ferlin A. The use of nutraceuticals in male sexual and reproductive disturbances: position statement from the Italian Society of Andrology and Sexual Medicine (SIAMS). J Endocrinol Invest 2017; 40(12): 1389-97.

CHAPTER 5

Energetic Anatomy and Physiology in Male Infertility

Abstract: The focus on fertility and to ensure offspring was a very important element in the Confucian tradition because of the practice of ancestor worship. Even in the Taoist tradition fertility was significant, since the practices for obtaining longevity and immortality used techniques in the area of sexuality and reproduction. The anatomy of the male genital tract in Chinese medicine uses specific terms for visible structures such as the external genitalia, while there are more functional and structural terms for some internal structures. The chapter also describes the relationships of the Organs and Channels with the male reproductive system and the energetics of the spermiogram. The term *zong jin* has been extensively commented upon, because its different layers of meaning can reveal a complex and fascinating approach to male sexual and reproductive functioning.

Keywords: Bao, Barrier of Essence, Chamber of Essence, Channels, Chong Mai, Cinnabar Field, Dai Mai, Dan Tian, Essence, Huangdi Neijing, Li Shizhen, Ling Shu, Ming Men, Ministerial Fire, Organs, Sperm Chamber, Su Wen, Tiangui, Zhen Jiu Jia Yi Jing, Zong Jin.

HISTORICAL BACKGROUND

In the early days of Chinese medicine, the body was not studied in its physical aspect but was regarded as a set of functions, focusing on the process rather than the structure [1]. *The Inner Classic of the Yellow Emperor* (*Huangdi Neijing*), an imaginary dialogue between the Yellow Emperor and the doctor Qibo, portrays the Emperor's body as the perfect body, where the phenomena of Heaven, Earth and Humankind can be studied and followed in their transformations in a cosmology that includes Qi, Yin, Yang and the five movements. In this cosmological view the body was basically androgynous, where Yin functions and Yang functions were in equilibrium, and the twelve meridians and the five elements were the same in both males and females. Similarly, in the reproductive aspect there was no difference between the sexes: reproduction was the domain of Kidney and Water, Yin in nature for both males and females. The same terms indicated the external genitalia (Yin Chu 陰處 - place of Yin, or Yin Qi

陰器 - instrument of Yin), and secondary sexual characteristics such as beard or breasts were disregarded. The only difference between male and female in the Internal Canon concerned the length of life cycles, cycles of eight years for men, associated with Yang and even numbers, and cycles of seven years for women, associated with Yin and odd numbers (*Su Wen* I: Chapter 3). Apart from the length, other aspects of the cycles were comparable, with similar events at puberty and at the end of the reproductive period: as in menopausal women menstrual blood decreases, so in andropausal men, semen decreases.

In the 7th century A.D. the separation between man and woman began with Sun Si Miao (581–682 AD), a distinguished physician of the Tang Dynasty and considered the "king of medicine". He presented for the first time some specific prescriptions for women in the treaty *"Beiji Qianjin Yaofang"* (*Prescriptions worth a thousand pieces of gold for every emergency*, completed in 652 AD) [2] In this treatise Sun Si Miao also discussed male infertility due to Jing deficiency.

The focus on fertility and to ensure offspring was a very important element in the Confucian tradition because of the practice of ancestor worship. Even in the Taoist tradition fertility was significant, since the practices for obtaining longevity and immortality used techniques in the area of sexuality and reproduction.

ANATOMY OF THE MALE GENITAL TRACT ACCORDING TO CHINESE MEDICINE

The anatomy of the male genital tract in Chinese medicine uses specific terms for visible structures as the external genitalia, while there are more functional and structural terms for some internal structures such as the Chamber of Essence (Jing Shi), the Barrier of Essence (Jing Guan), and the Seminal Way (Jing Dao).

The scrotum was called in many ways, including "bag of the Kidney" (Shen Nang) and "bag of the Yin" (Yin Nang), while the testes and epididymis, which were not separated in the pre-modern era, were called also "the seed of the Kidney" (Shen Zi) or "Marshy Ball" (Gao Wan, where Gao is the swamp and Wan is the ball of a blowgun).

The prostate was commonly called the "Room of the Essence" (Shi Jing). However, some texts, especially the Nan Jing, refer to the prostate as part of the Ming Men.

The vas deferens may be likened to the Seminal Way (Jing Dao), while there is no anatomical structure corresponding to the Barrier of the Essence. The Barrier of Essence (Jing Guan) is defined as "a gate that is felt to open on ejaculation" by

Zhang Jie-Bin (1563–1640). Signs such as seminal efflux (loss occurring day and night), seminal emission (loss at night), and premature ejaculation are attributed to "insecurity of the Essence gate" due to Kidney disease [3].

The Sperm Chamber is the male reproductive organ, whose function is to produce and store sperm. Like the uterus in women, it is the place where Qi and Blood converge to form the fetus. The Sperm Chamber is located in the lower Cinnabar Field (Dan Tian). Cinnabar is mercury sulphide, an extremely toxic substance, but it is also the alchemical philosopher's stone in the East as it allows the alchemical transformation to achieve immortality. There are three Cinnabar Fields in three different areas of the body. They are in different locations in men and in women, but one of them is always in the lower abdomen, a sign of the importance of this area in the process of alchemical transformation. The *Lao Zi Zhong Jing* (*Middle Classic of Lao Zi*) states: "The lower Cinnabar Field is the root of the human body, where Essence accumulates, and it is the place of origin of the five breaths (Qi of the five Organs). In man there is an accumulation of the Essence, in the woman of the menses."

The Sperm Chamber is also called Bao. Bao is a term whose ideogram is composed of the radical flesh and a part that has the sense of "entangled", hence the translation "envelope". It represents all bodies wrapped by or consisting of a membrane, such as the placenta, the bladder, the uterus, *etc.*, and refers to both men and women. It is often mistranslated as "uterus", which instead corresponds to the term "Zi Bao" (Seed Envelope). The character of Bao is the same as that used to refer to the Pericardium (Xin Bao). It is the place where Jing is accumulated and where the transformation of Qi and Blood happens. The "*Golden Mirror of Medicine*" (*Yi Zong Jin Jian*, 1742) states: "Ren Mai rises from the lower abdomen, externally from the abdomen, internally in the Bao (...) which is also called Dan Tian in both men and women: in women it is the uterus, in men it is the Sperm Chamber".

The Bao has a relationship with Ming Men, since Ming Men is the place where the envelope is attached. Bao also has a relationship with the Extraordinary Meridians, because the first generation Extraordinary Meridians originate from the Ming Men. Finally, Bao has a relationship with the Blood: the *Su Wen* I: cap. 33 talks about a communication between Heart and the uterus with a vase called "Bao Mai". Consequently, in the problems of Blood at the level of Bao, we must think also of the Heart, because all events affecting the emotions, of which the Heart is the support, can resonate with the Bao [4].

The male genital organ is the anterior orifice (*qian yin*) as opposed to the anus, the posterior orifice (*hou yin*), the two lower orifices (*xià qiào*) or turbid orifices (*zhuò qiào*) governed by the Kidney. It has been identified by several names: *jing* (stem), *yu jing* (jade stem), or *zong jin*.

It is worth spending some time on the term *zong jin*, because its different layers of meaning can reveal a complex and fascinating approach to male sexual and reproductive functioning.

In the *Ling Shu* (LS 13), the locomotor apparatus is described as being organized in twelve *Jing Jin* (tendino-muscular or sinew channels) and one *Zong Jin*. The *Jing Jin* represent a set of muscles from the periphery to the axial region and are often superimposed on the channel pathway, while the *zong jin* has an unclear role in the system.

Zōng 宗 has different meanings in the Ricci's dictionary (R5240), such as "temple of the ancestors; ancestors; clan; to respect; class, category; school, sect; master, head of school; foundation, fundamental, essential". *Zong* is the continuity and progress of the lineage, what is worthy of honour, important and venerable; what draws under its authority. It summarizes all the vital relationships of the individual with the environment and with others.

Jīn 筋 has the radical for bamboo in the upper part and the radical for flesh and the radical for power/strength in the lower part. Its meanings are: sinew (a tough, stringy, elastic part of the body); tendon, palpable muscle; a vein visible at the surface of the body; penis [5].

Zong jin has been usually translated as: ancestral sinew(s) or ancestral tendon/muscle, tendon/muscle of the ancestors, male external genitals, and confluence of tendons or gathering sinew. Together with the variety of translations there is also a variety of interpretations of what this term refers to, but first let's look at the original description of the *zong jin* in the *Huang Di Nei Jing Su Wen* in chapter 44:

The Yang brilliance [conduit] is the sea of the five depots and six palaces, it is responsible for keeping the basic sinew (*zong jin*) moist. The basic sinew is responsible for binding together the bones and for the free movement of the trigger joint. The thoroughfare vessel is the sea of the conduit vessels. It is responsible for pouring [liquid] into the ravines and valleys. It unites with the yang brilliance [conduit] at the basic sinew. The yin and the yang [conduits] are brought together at the meeting point with the basic sinew. This meeting takes place at the qi street, and the yang brilliance [conduit] is their chief. They are all connected with the belt vessel, and they are connected with the supervisor vessel. Hence, when the yang brilliance [conduit] is depleted, then the basic sinew slackens and the belt vessel fails to pull [tight]. Hence the feet suffer from limpness and do not function [6].

It is clear from this description that the *zong jin* is a strategic intersection of the Chong Mai (thoroughfare vessel), the Du Mai (supervisor vessel) and the Dai Mai (belt vessel) (anterior heaven) with the Stomach/Yang brilliance conduit (posterior heaven). These meridians influence a variety of muscle groups, but different commentators have given different interpretations of this relationship.

For Wang Bing, an important commentator of the Nei Jing from the 9th century CE, the *zong jin* is located above the pubis, goes up to the abdomen and chest, and passes down through the sacrum to move up along the back to the neck. The trigger joint for which the *zong jin* is responsible is the lower back in its bending and stretching movements, and the qi street refers to the locations on both sides of the pubic hair where the movement in the vessels can be felt. Other translators interpret the qi street as the point **ST30** Qichong, and identify higher and lower parts of the *zong jin* (the Yin and Yang channels = Chong mai and Stomach channel) which converge at Qichong (**ST30**).

Maciocia relates the term *zong jin* to the rectus abdominis and the erector spinae muscles and the penis, as they are controlled by the Stomach channel, the Penetrating vessel and the Governor vessel [7].

The Daoist approach includes different muscular structures in the definition of *zong jin*. For Jeffrey Yuen, *zong jin* can refer to either the genitals (the sinew responsible for creating posterity), the diaphragm (the muscle that connects us with the air which our ancestors breathed) or the abdominal rectus muscle (it influences the Middle Burner and descends to the genitals). According to Daoist teachings reported by Boggie, the *zong jin* is a set of five paired sinews whose primary function is to maintain the integrity and the functionality of the three bony cavities [8]. The muscles and tendons involved are the sternocleido-mastoideus muscle, the diaphragm, the iliopsoas muscle, the rectus abdominis muscle and the paravertebral and gluteal muscles, which can become a holding place for latent external and internal pathogenic factors. The latent pathogens can be eliminated by relaxing the sinews holding them, starting with the opening points of the *zong jin* (**GB41** Zulinqi and **GB27** Wushu).

A contemporary piece of research done on the conduits that are in relation with the *zong jin*, according to the Suwen, analysed the muscular indications of their points, showing that the *zong jin* controls the following muscles: rectus abdominis muscle (ST and KI), obliques and transverse muscles of the abdomen (GV), quadriceps femoralis muscle (ST), rotator muscles of the thigh (CV), gluteal muscles (Daimai and GV), lumbar muscles (CV and GV), latissimus dorsalis muscle (Daimai) [9] As a whole these muscles have no role in the upright posture in a static sense, but have an essential role in maintaining the balance and the standing position while walking, that is the upright posture in a dynamic sense. Thus the *zong jin* is a centre of movement because it is a convergence of tendons.

But why is the male genital organ associated with various muscle groups? What is the connection between the penis, and maintaining balance and the upright position while walking? Between the male genital organs and the centre and crossroads of all musculoskeletal apparatus?

A possible answer could come from Qigong, where there is one sequence which activates all the muscles of the *zong jin*. In this sequence the man lies down on the floor with the arms along the body, then raises his head and feels the tension in the abdominal muscles (activation of the sternocleidomastoideus and rectus abdominis muscles). Next he pulls the navel inside and then upside (activation of the transverse and obliquus muscles). In the last part he raises both legs and draws an infinity sign with both feet (activation of the gluteal and quadriceps muscles). The interesting part is that the activation of all the *zong jin* muscles in this qigong sequence has an indication to improve the male sexual and reproductive health!

It is then apparent that the term *zong jin* does not indicate either groups of muscles or the male external genitals. On the contrary, the ancient Chinese doctors had a very clear awareness of the integration of different body systems in male sexuality and fertility. In the West we have lost track of this, and we consider that the penis is separated from the rest of the body. This integrated view of the *zong jin* may explain why physical exercise is so important for good health and fertility.

Organs/Zang and Male Fertility

The Kidneys store the Essences, first Yuanqi, or original Qi of Former Heaven, and they also store the essences of Later Heaven, created by the transformation of the air, and of liquid and solid foods. In the classical system the Kidneys were associated with Water, but in the Song era this was replaced by the system of "five cycles and six Qi", in which the Kidneys were split into left Kidney, corresponding to Water, and right Kidney, corresponding to Ministerial Fire (Despeux & Hinrichs, 2012) [10]. The Ministerial Fire is the Yang engine of the body, and is a Fire that can generate Water, and that is inseparable and interdependent with Water. The Water of the Kidney is the Jing, which is converted into Yuan Qi to support the functions of the Organs and Bowels of the whole body. The Ministerial Fire is the original Yang of Former Heaven, whose purpose is to carry out orders of the Imperial Fire, that is the Heart [11]. These concepts are very important for the alchemical Taoist practices, which through the reversal and the union of opposites had to gather in the Middle Burner the Water coming down from the Heart and the Fire rising from the Kidneys.

The Ministerial Fire also originates from the Ming Men, the space between the two kidneys, which is located behind the navel or at three distances (cun) below the navel (**CV4**, Guanyuan) or at the second lumbar vertebra (**GV4**, Mingmen). Ming Men is the residence of the ancestral energies, the "Gate of Destiny". It is essential also for the evolution of the individual, from his or her growth in the uterus to life after birth, and is considered the place where the mechanisms related to sexuality and reproduction develop. The Nanjing in the 36th difficulty states that "The kidneys are two, but they are not both kidneys, the one on the left is the Kidney, the one on the right is the Ming Men. The Ming Men (the door of the mandate) is the place where Jing-Shen dwells, the place to which the original influences (Yuanqi) are linked."

At the Organ level, the Kidney is the support of all the energies and provides Jing energy (Essence); for this reason the points **BL23** (Sheshu) and **BL52** (Zhishi), linked to the Kidneys, are also called the Palace of Jing (Jing Gong). The other Organs in close relationship with the pelvic region are essentially the Liver and the Spleen, which are related to the Blood (Spleen produces it and Liver stores it). The Lung governs Qi, is the upper source of water and moves the Liquids. Along with the Large and Small Intestine, the Lung has a role in the pathophysiology of Fluids that form both semen and urine.

The Heart, especially from the point of view of male sexuality, is considered as a "higher Kidney". It influences many sexual functions through its connections with the Conception Vessel, Governing Vessel and Chong Mai. Another important connection between Heart and sexual function is through the Ministerial Fire of the Ming Men. The Ministerial Fire warms and nourishes the Sperm Chamber; when it is deficient the Sperm Chamber is cold and this may be associated with impotence or low libido; when the Ministerial Fire is in excess it rises upward and hits the Heart and the Pericardium. The Pericardium (Xin Bao) forms a sexuality centre located in the Upper Burner, while the Sperm Chamber forms a sexuality centre located in the Lower Burner. The coordination of these two centres controls sexuality in men, because the Heart and the Pericardium above and the Kidney Ministerial Fire below regulate the rise and descent of Fire and Water, and inhibit and nourish each other.

Primary and Secondary Meridians and the Male Genital Tract

The male genital tract is passed across by several primary and secondary meridians. In particular, all Yin meridians of the lower limb, including the divergent meridians, have a relationship with the genital organs. Also, the three Yin sinew meridians of the foot pass the genital system and are inserted in the lower part of the pelvis, in the region between **CV3** (Zhongji) and **CV4** (Guanyuan). Among the yang meridians, only those of the stomach and gall bladder are connected with the genitals. For a more detailed discussion on the energetic anatomy of the pelvis see "Principles of Chinese medical andrology" [12].

The internal and external trajectories of the Stomach Meridian converge at **ST30** (Qichong), where the divergent Stomach Meridian originates. In the *Zhen Jiu Jia Yi Jing* there is a reference to the relationship between the Zong Jin and **ST30**: "all Yin and Yang Meridians come together in the Zong Jin and continue to meet **ST30** (Qichong), and the Yang Ming Meridian is the largest among them. They are all surrounded by Dai Mai and join with the Governor Vessel." **ST30** is also the point of origin of Chong Mai, which is the Sea of Blood, and is also called Qijie (junction of Qi) to indicate the passage of Qi in the pelvic region. The sinew and divergent Stomach Meridians gather in the genitals before spreading into the abdomen, and help to maintain a normal genito-urinary function. On the Stomach Meridian there is a point, **ST29** (Guilai), traditionally considered useful for genital problems. It was shown that its stimulation with electroacupuncture increases the blood flow in the testicular arteries (Cakmak *et al.*, 2008) [13]. This is relevant, because many conditions associated with aging and infertility (varicocele, oligoasthenozoospermia, low testosterone levels, torsion of the spermatic cord, *etc.*) are associated with decreased blood flow to the testicles.

The Spleen Meridian goes up along the leg and enters the abdomen. On its way to the Spleen and Stomach it nourishes the abdominal tissues and organs, including the genitals. The sinew and divergent Spleen Meridians accumulate in the genitals. The point **SP21** (Dabao), point of origin of the second Spleen Luo, contains the ideogram Da (large), which correlates with the transition from Former Heaven to Later Heaven, with the creation and nourishment at the beginning of existence, hence the relationship with the Ming Men and the Bao (Brici, 2001) [14].

The Heart Meridian does not have a direct link with the male genitalia, but an indirect one, *via* the Kidney Meridian within the Shao Yin movement and *via* the extraordinary meridians Conception Vessel, Governing Vessel and Chong Mai. Conception Vessel and Governor Vessel have a profound influence on sexuality, from sexual desire and excitement to erection and ejaculation. Chong Mai among other things controls the zong muscles of the abdomen, including the penis (Zong Jin). Sexual dysfunctions in the male, such as impotence or premature ejaculation, are often treated with points of the Heart Meridian, because they are almost always due to a dysfunction of the Heart Fire (deficiency or excess) rather than to a Kidney deficiency.

One of the internal branches of the Bladder Meridian enters the body at the level of the second lumbar vertebra and makes contact with the Kidney and Bladder, helping to support the urinary, sexual and reproductive functions. Also the divergent and luo Meridians of the Bladder are in contact with the Kidney and Bladder. The Bladder Meridian, *via* the back Shu points, acts directly on the Kidneys and on the Lower Burner, increasing the number and viability of sperm. In fact many protocols for the treatment of male infertility include points like **BL23** (Shenshu) and **BL32** (Ciliao).

The Kidney Meridian, according to the *Systematic Classic of Acupuncture and Moxibustion* (*Zhen Jiu Jia Yi Jing*), is connected with the Governing Vessel, which in its course in men "follows the penis to the perineum". In addition, the *Ling Shu* (LS 38) describes the path of the lower branch of Chong Mai when it enters the "great luo" (Da luo) of the Kidney Meridian, presumably at the level of **KI4** (Dazhong), providing a link between these meridians. The Chong Mai joins the ancestral tendon (*Su Wen* I: Chap. 44), and this is another reason that justifies the use of the points of the Kidney Meridian to treat andrological problems.

The divergent Meridian of the Pericardium houses the three Burners *via* the Luo Meridians, and the connection to the Lower Burner has a particular relevance to andrology issues.

The Gall Bladder Meridian houses the Kidney Mu alarm point **GB25** (Jingmen), which is often included in protocols for male infertility due to Kidney Yang deficiency (Lyttleton, 2013) [15].

The Liver meridian has a close relationship with the male genitalia, as described in the *Su Wen* (SW31 and SW39), in the *Ling Shu* (LS 10 and LS 52), and *Zhen Jiu Jia Yi Jing* (chaps. 2 and 7). According to these texts the Liver Meridian surrounds, envelops, and forms a network around the genitals, joining the tendons before reaching the Liver organ. The *Ling Shu* (LS 10) states "the Liver Meridian joins the tendons and the tendons assemble at the genitals." This description reveals the link between Tendons and penis since the penis is also identified with the Zong Jin ("water of Essences ancestral" or "meeting of Tendons" or "acquired energy" depending on how the term Zong is translated). On the Liver Meridian is **LR5** (Ligou), a point that has a particular tropism for the external genitalia and dissipates Damp/Heat. The Luo Jueyin Meridian also has a direct relationship with the external genitalia.

Extraordinary Meridians and the Male Genital Tract

The Extraordinary Meridians regulate Energy transport and homeostasis, acting as deposits in case of excess and releasing it in case of scarcity, and eliminating perverse energies. They preferentially transport the ancestral Qi, which is correlated to creation in all its forms, including procreation. Extraordinary Meridians linked to the pelvis are those that originate from the Ming Men: Chong Mai, Conception Vessel, Governing Vessel and Dai Mai. According to the *Ling Shu* (LS 65) a vessel originates from the Ming Men and descends to the perineum (the Zong Jin area), reaching **CV1** (Huiyin). From there Chong Mai, Governor Vessel and Conception Vessel branch, and are enclosed by Dai Mai at waist level. The Ming Men is the site of the destiny of a person, and the first generation Extraordinary Meridians must protect and fulfil the mandate.

The deep origin of this group of Meridians reflects their function to regulate the most fundamental aspects of Qi. These Extraordinary Meridians are also called "first generation" as they are the first to lead the energetic, and then physical, development of the embryo. These Meridians are connected to Seas: Sea of Yang and Sea of Marrow with Governor Vessel, Sea of Yin and Sea of Qi with Conception Vessel, Sea of twelve meridians and Sea of Blood with Chong Mai, and Sea of the Ming Men with Dai Mai (Nan Jing, 28th difficulty).

The second-generation meridians are Qiao Mai and Wei Mai, which have a function of liaison and regulation of vital functions, and of adapting the body to space and time.

The Extraordinary Meridians are described in a fragmentary fashion in the classical texts. Li Shizhen in 1578 wrote their main systematic treatise called "Study of the eight extraordinary meridians," which has been commented on in recent times by Chace & Shima (2010) and has been summarized here [16].

Governor Vessel originates from deep within the pelvis, it surrounds the penis and at the perineum (**CV1**) it joins Conception Vessel, then goes up along the coccyx to connect with the Kidney and Bladder meridians and to the Kidney organ. Another branch goes up along the column and enters the Brain through the point **GV16** (Fengfu). Governor Vessel is also called the Sea of Yang because it is distributed mainly in the Yang region of the body and connects with all six Yang Primary Meridians at **GV14** (Dazhui). The ancient ideogram of Governor Vessel depicts a snake that coils around a man, an image common to many cultures which refers to the intrinsic power of the spinal column. In the embryo, Governor Vessel is responsible for the formation of the nervous system and for the cranio-caudal development. For this reason Governor Vessel is the Sea of Marrow, and regulates the Brain and Marrow pathophysiology and their relationship with the reproductive organs.

According to Li Shizhen, Governor Vessel is the axis that unifies the alchemical functions in the upper and lower portions of the body. In particular, the function of Governor Vessel is closely linked to the primordial void embodied in the lower abdomen, and both are the source of the primordial Yang, which can be awakened only in a state of perfect stillness and emptiness of mind.

Conception Vessel begins at **CV4** (Guanyuan), goes through **CV1** (Huiyin) and together with Governor Vessel passes through the coccyx and into the spine. It is distributed in the front (Yin) portion of the body and connects with all the Yin meridians, directly or indirectly, regulating all the Yin throughout the body. For this reason it is called the Sea of Yin. Passing the three Burners, Conception Vessel connects with all the Organs and Bowels, regulating their functions. The Luo Meridian of Conception Vessel is intertwined with Governor Vessel.

At the pelvic level, Conception Vessel distributes the Yin in the form of Blood, Yuan Qi and Fluids, and eliminates the Perverse factors that can be accumulated in the pelvis. According to the *Ling Shu* (LS 65), Conception Vessel and Chong Mai form the Sea of Meridians and of the small Luo collaterals, whose specific function is to feed the Zong Jin (in this case the penis).

Chong Mai originates from the area between the Kidneys together with Conception Vessel and Governor Vessel. According to the *Ling Shu* (LS 62), Chong Mai emerges at the level of **ST30** (Qichong) and spreads outward. It reaches **KI11** (Henggu, pubic bone), and continues along the pathway of the Kidney Meridian on the abdomen. It ends reaching the face, lips and mouth, while a branch passes to the spine and follows the pathway of the Governor Vessel. Another branch goes down to the sole of the foot. **ST30** is closely related to the acquired energy, while another point of Chong Mai, **CV4** (Guanyuan), is related to the ancestral energy. For this reason Chong Mai is the meridian that binds the Former Heaven to Later Heaven, it is at the crossroads representing the transition from potential to realization. **ST30** is also an area of great concentration of Qi and Blood, which plays a key role in the pelvic physiological functions.

Chong Mai is the first vessel that appears during embryonic life, with the task of distributing Yuanqi and innate Jing, necessary for the development of the embryo and fetus. The organizing function takes place thanks to the pair Chong Mai - Dai Mai; this pair of Extraordinary Meridians is responsible for organizing and structuring the reproductive function, as well as the functions of "entry into life" (chong = invasion, irruption, advance). Another relevant couple is Chong Mai - Conception Vessel, which contributes to the material (Chong Mai) and energetic (Conception Vessel) development of the genital organs and to their nutrition by the Blood. So Chong Mai has a pivotal role in all the sexual and genital reproductive physiology.

Another role of Chong Mai derives from the fact that it arises from the depth of the Ming Men. Some symptoms such as spermatorrhea could result from a Chong Mai disorder, due to an inability to hold Fluids and Blood which then escape outward. Other andrological symptoms related to Chong Mai are urethritis, genital edema and impotence.

According to Li Shizhen, the internal branch of Chong Mai passes through the anatomical location of the Yuan Qi, and in doing so it establishes a communication between Chong Mai, Triple Burner and Yuan Qi. In this way Chong Mai is an extension of the function of the Triple Burner to facilitate the dissemination of Yuan Qi, along with Conception Vessel and Governor Vessel. The key point is **SP4** (Gongsun). "Gong" is the grandfather of maternal origin and therefore it pertains to the Yin, the nourishment. Jeffrey Yuen states that **SP4** is in relationship with the ancestors and can be used for reproduction issues, needling it together with the points of the Kidney Meridian (with the needle pointing toward the midline).

The relationship with the Blood (Chong Mai is the "Sea of Blood") illustrates the connection between Chong Mai and some secondary sexual characteristics such as hair. According to the *Su Wen* (Chap. 17) "hair is the surplus of the Blood," and chap. 65 of the *Ling Shu* states: "When Blood (in Chong Mai) is sufficient, the Blood moistens the skin and makes the body hair." This explains why the Chong Mai constitution is associated with an alteration in the distribution of hair, up to full blown hirsutism. Women have a functional deficiency of Blood in the Chong Mai, while eunuchs have anatomical damage to Zong Jin (in this case the genitals) that damages Chong Mai and Conception Vessel; this is the reason why their cheeks are not nourished by the Blood and do not grow a beard.

The abnormalities of the extraordinary functions of Chong Mai are connected to the Blood and manifest themselves as depression, physical, psychological and sexual fatigue, sleep disturbances and sexual and/or reproductive problems. The symptoms occur mainly at the time of the "big changes" of life (*e.g.* puberty) and can be treated with **ST30** and **CV4**.

Dai Mai originates at **LR13** (Zhangmen) (confluence point of Spleen Meridian and Gall Bladder Meridian, Mu point of the Spleen Meridian), under the extremity of the tenth rib, and wraps around all meridians that pass in the trunk. It goes down in the lower abdominal region through the points **GB26** (Daimai), **GB27** (Weidao) and **GB28** (Wushu), and enters into a relationship with all the meridians, but for Li Shizhen it has a special relationship with the Kidney Meridian, because the divergent Kidney Meridian and Dai Mai are born one from the other, and Dai Mai could be seen as an extension the divergent Kidney Meridian. For this reason, Dai Mai influences the physiological functions of the body at the deepest levels.

Dai Mai also enters into connection with the Stomach Meridian and with Governor Vessel, and this is of particular importance for the nourishment of Zong Jin with Qi and Blood. During the embryonic period Dai Mai is in relationship with Zong Jin and connects the first structures of the embryo and organizes the development of Chong Mai.

Dai Mai is influenced mainly by the poor functioning of the Spleen. The link between Spleen, Dampness and Dai Mai, according to Li Shizhen, is evident in the key symptom of Dai Mai, that is leukorrhea in women. In men the equivalent consists of a "white excess". This derives from a weakening of Zong Jin (penis), caused by a deficiency of Spleen and Kidney Qi caused by obsessive persistent thoughts, excessive sexual activity, or frustration. The white colour of the excess is not due to Cold invasion, according to Li Shizhen, but is an expression of Damp/Heat and should be treated with moxa on **LR13** (Zhangmen), which Li identifies as the Mu point of Dai Mai. Another white excess can also be composed of seminal emission, in this case the point to be treated is **GV20** (Baihui).

Yin and Yang Qiao Mai develop in the embryo when the limbs start to grow. They regulate Yin and Yang all over the body, in particular the passage of Yin and Yang from the outside to the inside and back in the nictemeral rhythm. They are related to the upright posture and are responsible for social life (with the eyes, brain and legs that they cross), also through the regulation of the sleep-wake cycle.

Zhang Boduan, Buddhist, Confucian and Taoist scholar of the Song Dynasty, in the *"Classic of the Eight Meridians"* quoted by Li Shizhen states that Yin Qiao Mai is located in front of the perineum under the scrotum, and Yang Qiao Mai behind the perineum in the sacrococcygeal region [16]. This pathway, which is not described in the strictly medical texts like the Neijing and Nanjing, is related to the spiritual and energetic alchemical cultivation techniques, and from this perspective the Extraordinary Meridians are "hidden spirits", inaccessible and closed unless they have been deliberately activated. Yin Qiao Mai in this perspective has a fundamental role, since it must be the first to be activated, and even the Extraordinary Meridians of the first generation are subordinate to it. In this tradition the meridian Yin Qiao is called by various names: the Root of Heaven, the Door of Death, the Passage of Resurrection, *etc.* Its importance lies in the fact that it connects the Brain (upper cinnabar field) with **KI1** (Yongquan), and that its location in the perineum is in relation to the alchemical location of the cinnabar field. According to Zhang Boduan the field of cinnabar is near **CV1** (Huiyin) and the Divine Turtle (Ling Gui, *i.e.* the penis). Commenting on these different trajectories Li Shizhen states that the doctor must first experience in him- or herself the activity of Extraordinary Meridians through meditation, before using them in clinical practice.

Yin and Yang Wei Mai respectively bind all Yin and Yang Meridians and regulate Yin and Yang in the external part of the body. The 28th Difficulty of Nan Jing describes the Wei meridians as "bound like a network to the body", referring to their function to bind the body in an integrated unit. Yang Wei moves all the Yang and controls the defensive energy on the surface, while Yin Wei controls the nourishing energy deeper in the body. In andrology this leads to the regulation and harmonization of Yin and Yang in the body, including the pelvis.

PATHOPHYSIOLOGY OF MALE INFERTILITY

Male fertility and sperm are ruled by the Kidneys. The Kidneys store the Jing (the essential Qi, which roughly corresponds to the modern concept of male and female gametes), and are at the root of sexual development, of libido and of fertility, and control the urethra and the testicles. When there is enough Kidney Qi, Jing and sperm can be produced. Kidney Yang serves to disperse and activate: it controls sexual activity, hormone secretion, and is the principle of reproduction. Kidney Yang regulates erection, ejaculation and the movement of sperm to the oocyte. Kidney Yin is the source of sperm, it can nourish and facilitate the production of sperm, so sperm quality and quantity depend on Kidney Yin.

The Liver is closely connected to the Kidney, and its deep and lasting root is the Kidney Yang (Fire of Ming Men), which is transferred to the Liver at puberty. The Liver governs the tendons (the penis corresponds to Zong Jin "fundamental tendon") and Liver Fire can suddenly awaken the Zong Jin and start an erection. Maintenance of erection and swelling instead depend on Kidney Qi. Other organs are involved, because the size of the penis depends on Spleen Qi, and blood flow to the penis depends on Heart Qi.

A fertile man must have an adequate amount of Jing, the fire of his Ming Men must be sufficiently hot as to promote the generation and transformation of Kidney Jing into semen and sperm, he must have freely flowing Liver Qi to regulate the transformation of Kidney Qi and to maintain a normal ejaculatory function, he must be free of obstructions caused by Phlegm and Blood stasis so that the semen pathway is sufficiently open to allow normal ejaculation, he must be free of Damp-Heat and Heat toxins in the Sperm Chamber that could otherwise burn the seed and damage sperm, and he must have an adequate amount of Qi and Blood to ensure the constant cultivation of the essence of Later Heaven, that can be stored in the Kidney and which can replenish the essence of Former Heaven. If two or more of these physiological aspects are altered, the man becomes infertile.

ENERGETICS OF THE SPERMIOGRAM

The seminal fluid can be examined according to a Chinese energetic perspective, regarding it as a physical manifestation of the Essence. From a broader perspective, sexual desire is a function and a manifestation of Kidney Yang, while the sexual fluids, such as semen in men, are a manifestation of the Kidney Yin. In a closer perspective, the liquid part of the seminal fluid, watery and nutritious, represents the Yin component of the spermiogram, while the sperm, mobile and dynamic, represents the Yang component.

A deficiency of Kidney Yang leads to a seed that has no ability to reproduce. The subject has difficulty with ejaculation and the seed has low sperm motility.

A deficiency of Kidney Yin instead leads to the production of low amounts of seminal fluid, with a high teratogenesis.

If the semen is yellow and thickened, this indicates the presence of Heat or Excess.

CONSENT FOR PUBLICATION

Not applicable.

CONFLICT OF INTEREST

The author (editor) declares no conflict of interest, financial or otherwise.

ACKNOWLEDGEMENT

Declared none.

FURTHER READING

Di Stanislao C, De Berardinis D, Corradin M. Visceri e Meridiani. CEA 2012.

Hammer LI. The Extraordinary Acupuncture Meridians: Homeostatic Vessels. Am J Acup 1980; 8(2): 123–46.

Lomuscio A. I meridiani straordinari Qi Jing Ba Mai. Available from: http://www.albertolomuscio.it/AGOPUNTURA/MERIDIANI/Meridiani-Curiosi.pdf

Maciocia G. Men's sexual and prostate problems in Chinese Medicine. The Three Treasures Newsletters, Autumn 2005. Available from: http://www.threetreasures.com/newsletters/autumn05.html

Matsumoto K, Birch S, Felt R. Extraordinary Vessels. Taos, NM: Paradigm Publications 1986.

BIBLIOGRAPHY

[1]   Furth C. A Flourishing Yin: Gender in China's Medical History. Oakland, CA: University of California Press 1999.

[2]   Wilms S. Ten Times More Difficult to Treat. Female Bodies from Early Imperial China. Nan Nu 2005; 7(2): 182-215.
       [http://dx.doi.org/10.1163/156852605775248685]

[3]   Wiseman N, Feng Y. A Practical Dictionary of Traditional Chinese Medicine. Taos, NM: Paradigm Publications 1998.

[4]   Visconti S. L'energetica della pelvi Available from: http://webhtml.agopuntura.org/html/mandorla/rivista/numeri/Giugno_1998/pelvi.htm

[5]   Wiseman N, Feng Y. A Practical Dictionary of Traditional Chinese Medicine. Taos, NM: Paradigm Publications 1998.

[6]   Unschuld PU, Tessenow H. Huang Di Nei Jing Su Wen. An Annotated Translation of Huang Di's Inner Classic – Basic Questions: 2 volumes, Volumes of the Huang Di Nei Jing Su Wen Project. Oakland, CA: University of California Press 2011; pp. 661-3.

[7]   Maciocia G. The Channels of Acupuncture. London: Churchill Livingstone 2006.

[8]   Boggie L. Zong Jin: The Ancestral Sinews. Am J Tradit Chin Vet Med 2010; 5(2): 87-92.

[9]   Lafont JL. Les tendons des meridiens Tradition et modernite Available from: http://www.gera.fr/Downloads/Formation_Medicale/Meridiens-donnees-traditionnelles/Meridie-s-tendino_musculaires/lafont-120678.pdf

[10]   Despeux C, Hinrichs TJ. Asia India Americhe—La scienza in Cina (epoca Song-Yuan) Cap. 35: La Medicina Storia della Scienza, Enciclopedia Treccani 2012. Available from: http://www.treccani.it/enciclopedia/la-scienza-in-cina-l-epoca-song-yuan-la-medicina_%28Storia-della-Scienza%29/

[11]   Sionneau P. Regarding the Lower Origin of the Wei Qi Available from: http://sionneau.com/files/Regarding%20the%20Lower%20Origine%20of%20the%20Wei%20Qi.pdf

[12]   Damone M. Principles of Chinese medical andrology: An Integrated Approach to Male Reproductive & Urological Health. Boulder, CO: Blue Poppy Press 2008.

[13]   Cakmak YO, Akpinar IN, Ekinci G, Bekiroglu N. Point- and frequency-specific response of the testicular artery to abdominal electroacupuncture in humans. Fertil Steril 2008; 90(5): 1732-8.
       [http://dx.doi.org/10.1016/j.fertnstert.2007.08.013] [PMID: 18076881]

[14]   Brici P. Da il Grande La Mandorla Giugno 2001. Available from: http://www.agopuntura.org /wp-content/uploads/2015/05/LaMandorla-2011-06.pdf

[15]   Lyttleton J. Treatment of Infertility with Chinese Medicine. London: Churchill Livingstone 2013.

[16]   Chace C, Shima M. An Exposition on the Eight Extraordinary Vessels: Acupuncture, Alchemy, and Herbal Medicine. Seattle, WA: Eastland Press 2010.

CHAPTER 6

Traditional Chinese Medicine in Male Infertility

Abstract: Treatment with TCM offers many treatment options that can be tailored to the individual subject based on the symptoms and signs present, and the imbalance to be treated. The main TCM syndromes present in male infertility are described.

Keywords: Damp-Heat, Dampness, Deficiency, Empty Heat, Excess, Heart Blood, Jing, Kidney Qi, Kidney Yang, Kidney Yin, Liver Qi, Lower Burner, Phlegm, Pulse, Rehmannia, Shen, Spleen Qi, Stagnation, Stasis, Tongue.

The key Organ in male fertility according to Traditional Chinese Medicine (TCM) is the Kidney, because of its function of preserving the essence and governing reproduction. If Kidney Qi and Yin are sufficient, the man can generate. In this role, the Kidney is assisted by the Liver, the Heart and the Spleen.

Male infertility may be associated with many TCM syndromes with Deficiency or Excess, Heat or Cold, with problems of Qi or Blood, or imbalances of Yin and Yang. In most cases there is an underlying Kidney deficiency, which according to TCM is also present in the Excess forms, fostered by an underlying Kidney deficiency or its complications. The Spleen may be involved in the pathogenesis of infertility when its functions of transportation and transformation are deficient, resulting in the formation of Dampness and Phlegm. The Liver ensures a harmonious flow of Qi when it is not burdened with emotional problems, while the stagnation of Liver Qi, which evolves into Liver Fire, may consume the water of the Kidney, inhibiting the passage of sperm. Stress can damage the Heart, particularly Heart Qi and Blood, causing infertility.

Traditionally the description of each specific TCM syndrome includes its etiology. For example, Empty syndromes are typically the result of stress and an exhausting life style, while Excess syndromes are related to Qi or Blood stagnation, or accumulation of Damp-Heat. However, the causal relationship need not be unequivocal or proved in order to start the treatment.

This is a difference between Chinese medicine and Western medicine, so if a person has a syndromic picture but does not report a history of the traditional causes of this syndrome, he/she is treated anyway according to the syndrome that emerges from the assessment.

Treatment with TCM offers many treatment options that can be tailored to the individual subject based on the symptoms and signs present and the imbalance to be treated. Several authors discuss the treatment of male infertility, see for example Di Stanislao 2004, Lyttleton 2004, Damone 2008, Deadman 2008, and Chen and Li 2008.

LIFESTYLE MODIFICATIONS

TCM can contribute to the treatment of male infertility not only with acupuncture and Chinese pharmacology, but also with advice on lifestyle.

A regular sexual activity maintains the free flow of Qi, Blood and Jing, and thus it maintains fertility. The longer the sperm remains in the Bao and testes, the longer the risk that it will be damaged by toxic Heat, Dampness, Phlegm and Blood stasis. On the other hand, excessive sexual activity can damage the Essence and lead to infertility through other mechanisms. Recommendations have been made on how to practise healthy sexual activity starting from the *Inner Canon of the Yellow Emperor*. For example, it is better to abstain if intoxicated, sweaty or after cold exposure, so as not to deplete Jing. In the *Prescriptions worth a thousand pieces of gold for every emergency (Beiji Qianjin Yaofang)* Sun Simiao recommended not to take medicines and tonics to promote sexuality if less than 40 years old, so as not to exhaust the Jing and Marrows. Other conditions in which it is better to abstain from sexual activity are at a full moon or new moon, during a storm, before having digested a heavy meal, after great efforts, with wet hair or after a tiring journey or before the healing of a drained wound (Noll & Wilms, 2009) [1].

Since Heat and its toxins damage the sperm, it is necessary to treat underlying causes that can generate the toxic Heat. In terms of Western medicine this corresponds to treating any infection or inflammation that is present in the body, from chronic prostatitis to sexually transmitted infections to pharyngitis and periodontal abscesses.

In the theory of the Three Treasures (Shen, Qi and Jing), to generate the Essence the Shen must be abundant and harmonious. So, men suffering from infertility should be encouraged to not repress their emotions, in order that their Liver and Heart Qi can flow freely.

Diet has a fundamental part in the treatment. It must be balanced and light, rich in vegetables and fruits, legumes, with small amounts of lean meat and fish. Large amounts of fatty, sweet and spicy foods must be avoided. A light diet increases the flow of Qi and Blood to the penis, it nourishes the Organs and Bowels and it prevents the accumulation of Dampness, Phlegm and Heat. Spicy foods may be beneficial in moderation, particularly in cold climates and in men with a constitutional Yang deficiency, as they can improve sperm motility and spermatogenesis. Excessive use of spicy foods, however, can drain the Essence and lead to the formation of Heat that consumes the Kidney Yin and Jing, damaging sperm and leading to infertility.

KIDNEY YIN DEFICIENCY

Kidney Yin is the root of the Yin of the body and is the source of semen. It helps the development of semen by increasing the quantity and improving the quality. Kidney Yin is damaged if people have a very stressful life, work for very long hours and go to sleep late, if they abuse substances *etc.*

The Kidney Yin vacuity does not retain the Yang, which escapes upwards and generates empty Heat. This in turn influences the Fluids, so it manifests itself with thickened and sticky seminal fluid, and a decrease in seminal volume and liquefaction. The increase in temperature will damage the sperm, causing oligozoospermia and teratozoospermia. The libido is increased but "empty", associated with anxiety, irritability, and poor sexual performance. There may be premature ejaculation and wet dreams with erotic dreams. Other general manifestations include restless sleep, many dreams, intolerance to light, dry mouth, dry throat, slight fever or feeling feverish, vertigo, tinnitus, memory loss, heaviness of the hips and knees, heat in the five centres, oliguria with dysuria, dark urine, constipation.

The Tongue is red with a thin coating, the Pulse is Fine (Xi) and, in the presence of empty Heat, also Rapid (Shuo). Sometimes the Kidney Yin deficiency manifests itself only with mild sleep disorders and reddened tongue tip. The pulse may be normal, particularly in athletic subjects.

Basic Prescriptions:

- *Wu Zi Yan Zong Wan* (Five Seed Progeny Pill, or Five Ancestors Pill) and *Zuogui Wan* (Restore the Left Pill): these formulae supplement and tonify the Yin, and invigorate the Jing and Kidneys. They are appropriate for most infertile men, because they tonify without overheating and nourish without overloading.
- *Liu Wei Di Huang Wan* (Six ingredient Pill with Rehmannia): nourishes Kidney Yin and secondly the Liver Yin, without purifying Empty Heat.

- ***Zhi Bai Di Huang Wan*** (Anemarrhena, Phellodendron and Rehmannia Pill): nourishes Kidney Yin and clears Empty Heat.

Acupuncture:

to nourish Yin: **SP6** (Sanyinjiao), **CV12** (Zhongwan), **KI3** (Taixi); to purify Empty Heat: **PC8** (Laogong), **HT8** (Shaofu), **LR2** (Xingjian); **CV4** (Guanyuan), **GV4** (Mingmen), **BL23** (Shenshu), **BL52** (Zhishi), **KI2** (Rangu), **KI6** (Zhaohai), **HT6** (Yinxi), **ST27** (Daju). **KI7** (Jiaoxin) is a point that is indicated to invigorate Kidney Yang, in this case it is used because it mobilizes the stagnant Yin.

KIDNEY YANG DEFICIENCY

Traditionally this syndrome is described as a consequence of excessive sexual activity and/or frequent masturbation, even if occurring only during adolescence. The sexual act disperses seminal fluid, which contains valuable Tiangui, direct manifestation of Kidney Jing, and it also disperses Kidney Qi. With time the deficiency of these substances will exhaust Kidney Yang. Nowadays stress can be practically considered an "equivalent" of sexual excesses. Yang deficiency can also result from chronic diseases and prolonged stagnation of External Cold, that damages the body's Yang.

Kidney Yang is the source of reproduction, it controls sexual intercourse (both penile erection and the ejaculation of semen), the movement of the sperm to the oocyte and hormonal secretion. It heats the Bao (Sperm Chamber) in the pelvis, supporting sexual function and reproductive health; without Kidney Yang the Bao becomes cold, so there will be general coldness especially in the lumbar region, psychophysical asthenia, back pain or weak loins, polyuria with clear urine. On a sexual level there is low libido, erectile difficulties up to impotence, weak ejaculation, low intensity orgasm, cold genitals.

The semen is watery and cold, with asthenozoospermia and/or prolonged time of liquefaction. There can be spermatorrhea and premature ejaculation. A typical symptom of Kidney Yang deficiency is early morning diarrhea; diarrhea after eating is related to the Spleen. Other symptoms and signs are apathy, fatigue, pallor, no desire to talk, weak lower back and knees, clear and abundant urine, aversion to cold, cold loins. The symptoms of aversion to cold and chilliness in Yang deficiency improve with exposure to warmth, unlike the invasion of pathogenic Cold, whose symptoms do not improve with exposure to warmth.

The Tongue is pale, moist, sometimes swollen, with thin and whitish coating, the Pulse is weak (Ruo) and Deep (Chen).

Basic Prescriptions:

- *You Gui Wan* (Restore the Right Kidney Pill) modified by the addition of *He Shou Wu* (Radix Polygoni Multiflori).
- *Jin Gui Shen Qi Wan* (Kidney Qi Pill from the Golden Cabinet): tonifies and warms the Kidney Yang.
- *Gui Ling Ji* (Tortoise Age Placenta Pill) for Kidney Yang deficiency and depletion of the Fire of Ming Men. If there is sexual dysfunction, *San Qi* (Radix pseudoginseng) or *Dan Shen Wan* (Four-Miracle Pill) can be added.

Acupuncture:

With needles and moxa treat: **BL23** (Shenshu), **GV4** (Mingmen), **KI3** (Taixi), **KI 7** (Fuliu), **CV6** (Qihai); **GB25** (Jingmen), **BL30** (Baihuanshu), **KI2** (Rangu), **KI12** (Dahe), **CV2** (Qugu), **BL52** (Zhishi).

KIDNEY QI DEFICIENCY

The Kidney is the root of congenital Qi, Jing and Blood, and is the basis for development, growth and reproduction. When Kidney Qi is sufficient, it can produce Jing and semen. Kidney Qi is formed when Kidney Yang vaporizes Kidney Yin, so its deficiency follows from a deficiency of either Kidney Yin or Kidney Yang, and can manifest with symptoms of both conditions.

Signs of deficiency of Kidney Qi include spermaturia and oligozoospermia; in general there will be weakness and soreness in the lower back and knees, nocturia, fatigue, physical and mental fatigue, pale skin.

The Tongue is pale with thin white coating, the Pulse Deep (Chen) and Fine (Xi).

Basic Prescriptions:

- *Shen Bao* (Kidney's Treasure): tonifies Kidney Yin, Kidney Yang, Kidney Qi and Kidney Jing
- *Shen Qi Da Bu Wan* (Great Ginseng and Astragalus Tonifying Pill): tonifies Qi.

Acupuncture:

With the technique of warm needle (moxa on needle): **GV4** (Mingmen), **GV20** (Baihui), **KI2** (Rangu), **KI3** (Taixi), **KI6** (Zhaohai), **CV6** (Qihai), **BL52** (Zhishi), **BL23** (Shenshu).

KIDNEY JING DEFICIENCY

The prenatal Jing forms the material basis of growth and fertility of the individual.

It becomes Kidney Qi and, when this is sufficient, the Tiangui can flow in the Conception Vessel and Chong Mai. The Jing can mature only when these two meridians are full, for then women begin to menstruate, and men begin to produce semen. At this time sexual activity can be fertile. When there is a deficiency of the Yin energy of Earlier Heaven, that is, the Jing, the Minister Fire of the Triple Burner starts moving with symptoms corresponding to Heat.

A congenital Jing deficiency can occur if the parents are too young, or if they have too many children, particularly if the parents are relatives, and can be associated with poor development of the secondary sexual characteristics, with underdeveloped testes or with chronic lack of interest in sex. The seminal fluid may have a decreased volume and oligozoospermia. If the Kidney Jing deficiency is acquired (Later Heaven), it may be associated with premature aging. This can happen after a prolonged illness, with Spleen Qi deficiency or Liver Blood deficiency, and with stress, which damages the Spleen and Stomach. Both Jing deficiencies, congenital or acquired, cause infertility that may be associated with genetic problems.

Other signs and symptoms include bone pain, cold to the bones, fatigue, weakness, loss of memory and difficulty concentrating. When the Jing deficiency leads to Empty Heat, there will be hot flashes and night sweats.

The Tongue is small (in width), thin (in thickness) and without coating, the Pulse is Deep (Chen), Weak (Ruo), and Empty (Xu).

Basic Prescriptions:

- *Gou qi zi* (Fructus Lycii) 15g: eat in the evening for two months.
- *Wu Zi Yan Zong Wan* (Five Seed Progeny Pill, or Five Ancestors Pill): to be used if there is teratozoospermia. It has a strong antioxidant effect and it increases levels of testosterone [2] It can also be added to the treatment strategies of Yin and Yang deficiencies.
- *Nan Xing Bu Shen Fang* (Men's Tonify Kidney Pill) for abnormalities in the spermiogram.

Acupuncture:

KI3 (Taixi), **KI6** (Zhaohai), **CV4** (Guanyuan), **GV4** (Mingmen), **GV16** (Fengfu), **GV20** (Baihui), **BL11** (Dazhu), **BL23** (Shenshu), **BL43** (Gaohuangshu), **GB39** (Xuanzhong).

DEFICIENCY OF SPLEEN QI AND HEART BLOOD

The Spleen is the Later Heaven and the root of acquired Jing. It nourishes the

Kidneys and, in the case of Spleen deficiency, both Yin and Yang Kidneys can go into deficiency. Spleen deficiency causes a deficiency of Qi, which may result in a weak ejaculation: the Spleen is related to the muscles, and in TCM the prostate is a muscle. The decrease in the force of contraction of the prostate can be so severe that it leads to the inability to ejaculate; furthermore with Qi deficiency the movement of sperm cannot be activated, because the progressive motility of sperm depends on Yang and Qi.

Spleen deficiency causes deep depression, pallor, generalized feeling of heaviness, shortness of breath with little desire to talk, digestive difficulties and postprandial bloating, loose stools, fatigue and weak muscles, poor appetite. Poor appetite is also defined as desire to eat but, in front of a full refrigerator, you do not know what to choose. Sexual desire is minimal and the ejaculate is watery and thin. The presence of anti-sperm antibodies can be associated with Spleen Qi deficiency.

The picture can be complicated by Heart and Liver Blood deficiency, which then present with insomnia, palpitations, dizziness, *etc.*, and by Dampness, which can cause relapsing fungal infections.

The Tongue is pale with thin coating, sometimes swollen with teeth marks, the Pulse is Deep (Chen) and/or Fine (Xi).

Basic Prescriptions:

- ***Ba Zhen Sheng Jing Tang*** (Eight Treasures Decoction to promote Jing). The decoction tonifies and supplements Qi, harmonizes and tonifies the Middle Burner, supplements Blood and tonifies Jing.
- ***Ren Shen Gui Pi Wan*** (Ginseng and Longan Pill): calms the mind, nourishes the Heart, tonifies Spleen, Qi and Blood.

Acupuncture:

Also using moxa, treat: **BL15** (Xinshu), **BL20** (Pishu), **ST36** (Zusanli), **HT7** (Shenmen).

LIVER QI STAGNATION

Liver Qi Stagnation is caused by a lack of physical activity, prolonged sitting, and especially Internal Pathogenic Factors, in particular excessive sadness and repression of emotions.

Smooth flowing of Liver Qi also affects the secretion and ejaculation of sperm. When the man is depressed and the Liver loses its function of spreading Qi, the force of ejaculation is decreased, sometimes up to an inability to ejaculate. The Liver governs the tendons, and the penis is sometimes identified as the "Zong Jin" (also translated as "meeting of 100 tendons"). When there is Liver Qi stagnation there can be also a weak erection.

Other symptoms and signs include intercostal and flank tension, chest tightness, shortness of breath, a sensation of a lump in the throat, belching, frequent sighs, basically depressed attitude, mood swings, irritability, suppressed anger. In the genital area there can be incomplete erection, painful ejaculation, and hemospermia. In the long run Liver Qi stagnation can evolve into Blood stasis, with varicocele, masses, *etc*.

The Tongue tends to be of normal colour, the Pulse is Tight (Jin) or Wiry (Xian).

Basic Prescription:

• *Xiao Yao San* (Free and Easy Wanderer Powder): harmonizes Liver and Spleen, nourishes Liver Blood, calms Liver Qi and invigorates Spleen Qi.

Acupuncture:

Long treatment sessions (at least 30 minutes) treat in dispersion: **BL18** (Ganshu), **LR2** (Xingjian), **LR3** (Taichong), **BL17** (Geshu); **BL20** (Pishu) if there is a white film on the tongue, as a sign of Liver inhibiting the Spleen; **CV1** (Huiyin) and **CV2** (Qugu) increase the circulation of Qi and Blood in the genitals, while **ST30** (Qichong) and **BL31** (Shangliao) remove the stagnation in the Lower Burner.

LIVER BLOOD STASIS

Blood Stasis of the Liver is often a consequence of Liver Qi Stagnation or of the action of Internal Pathogenic Factors. Other causes include testicular trauma and infections of the genital tract.

The semen will present an increase in the time of liquefaction and various anomalies like oligozoo-azoospermia, asthenozoospermia, hematospermia or teratozoospermia. Varicocele is a key sign, and it can be associated with excruciating pain on ejaculation, abdominal pain (especially at night), and dark complexion or purple nails, lips and/or skin.

The Tongue is dark red to purple, sometimes with ecchimoses on the sides, the Pulse is Wiry (Xian), Deep (Chen) and Choppy (Se), or Fine (Xi) and Choppy (Se).

Basic Prescription:

• *Xue Fu Zhu Yu Tang* (Drive Out Stasis in the Mansion of Blood Decoction). The decoction moves the Blood, disperses the Stasis, and restores the path of the ejaculate. For best results it should be combined with formulas that disperse, heat, tonify or move Blood, according to the constitution and the presenting syndrome of the man.

Acupuncture:

To dissolve the Stasis the following acupoints are bled with a lancet or a plum blossom hammer: **SP6** (Sanyinjiao), **SP10** Xuehai), **LR5** (Ligou), **BL32** (Ciliao), **CV4** (Guanyuan), **BL17** (Geshu).

DAMP-HEAT ACCUMULATION IN THE LOWER BURNER

Damp/Heat can arise because of dietary excesses (in particular the excesses of greasy and spicy foods, smoking and drinking), after previous unresolved infections (prostatitis, cystitis, sexually transmitted diseases such as gonorrhea, *etc.*), or in the presence of Liver-Spleen disharmony, Kidney Yin deficiency with Empty Heat, Yang Kidney deficiency which does not metabolize Dampness, or constitutional Yang hyperactivity that heats and thickens the Fluids. If the Dampness cannot be metabolized by the Spleen and Stomach, it goes down to the Lower Burner, causing Qi stagnation, liberation of Heat and condensation of Dampness, which manifest themselves as inflammation (Heat) and obstructions (Dampness).

Local genitourinary signs include acute inflammations like balanoposthitis, urethritis, cystitis, prostatitis and prostatovescicolitis; the pivotal sign is abnormal penile discharge. The external genitals are moist, sometimes with scrotal eczema. Urination is difficult, painful, scanty or turbid, and is followed by losses from the urethral meatus and itching or pain in the penis. There may be dark urine and spermaturia.

There can be premature or delayed ejaculation, or erection without ejaculation, with testicular swelling and discomfort after intercourse. The ejaculate is yellowish (leucospermia and pus) or reddish (hemospermia), and there is an absence of liquefaction, oligozoospermia, teratozoospermia *etc.*

At the systemic level there can be anxiety, irritability, bitter mouth, halitosis, desire to drink cold drinks, thirst without desire to drink, feeling of chest and epigastric fullness, heaviness of the legs and head. The feces will be wet, smelly and sticky and difficult to evacuate.

This condition can evolve towards the formation of Toxic Heat (Du), which burns and thickens the Blood. The manifestations include the formation of testicular or scrotal abscess from Blood stasis.

The Tongue has a yellow, thickened and sticky coating, the Pulse is rapid (Shuo) and Slippery (Hua) and/or Wiry (Xian).

Basic Prescriptions:

- *Bei Xie Shen Shi Tang* (Dioscorea Hypoglauca Decoction to Eliminate Dampness): if Heat prevails.
- *Bei Xie Fen Qing Yin* (Dioscorea Hypoglauca Decoction to Separate the Clear): if Dampness prevails.
- *Long Dan Xie Gan Tang* (Gentian Drain Fire Decoction): in the presence of signs of Liver involvement (red eyes, headache, irritability, *etc.*).

Acupuncture:

CV3 (Zhongji), **SP9** (Yinlinquan), **LR2** (Xingjian), **LR5** (Ligou) (with needles and cupping). These points can be added: **CV4** (Guanyuan), **KI7** (Fuliu), **KI10** (Yingu), **BL35** (Huiyang), **CV1** (Huiyin), **LR8** (Ququan), **SP6** (Sanyinjiao) and **SP7** (Lougu). **BL27** (Xiaoshangshu) and **BL28** (Pangguangshu) can be used to treat genital discharge.

PHLEGM AND BLOOD STASIS BLOCKING THE PASSAGE OF ESSENCE

A constitutional Spleen Qi deficiency and the excessive consumption of fatty and sugary foods can unbalance the Spleen's ability to transport and transform, particularly in overweight and obese men. This causes Dampness and Food Stasis, which eventually condense into Phlegm. Phlegm in turn blocks the passage of Essence and forms a significant obstruction to the normal male sexual and reproductive function. The signs include seminal alterations like decreased semen volume, oligozoospermia, inability to ejaculate and teratozoospermia.

Phlegm is a cause of obstruction to the movement and transformation of other Yin aspects of the body, and thus it can lead to Blood stasis. The combination of Phlegm and Blood stasis is described as "mutual bond of Phlegm and Blood stasis" or "Phlegm stasis" (tan yu). Blood stasis can originate from Phlegm stasis, but it can also be formed independently of this mechanism by the dehydrating action of the Heat on the Blood, or after traumas and surgeries. The signs of Blood stasis are epistaxis, petechiae, hemospermia, fixed and persistent stabbing pains, presence of fixed abdominal masses, purple lips and complexion. Blood stasis in the pelvis can cause scrotal tenderness and/or heaviness but also stabbing pain. Microcirculatory disorders, obstruction of the seminiferous ducts and varicocele are part of this syndrome.

The Tongue is dark red to purple, the Pulse is Wiry (Xian).

Basic Prescription:

- *Cang Fu Dao Tan Tang* (Atractylodes and Cyperus Decoction to Expel Phlegm): dries Dampness, transforms accumulated Phlegm, moves Qi, eliminates stagnation.

Acupuncture:

SP10 (Xuehai), **LR5** (Ligou), **BL32** (Ciliao), **CV4** (Guanyuan) and **BL17** (Geshu) (with needles and plum blossom hammer). Secondary points: **SP6** (Sanyinjiao), **ST30** (Qichong), **BL31** (Shangliao), **LR1** (Dadun).

GENERAL TREATMENT

Often a man suffering from infertility does not present a clear syndromic picture according to the principles of TCM. In these cases, the appearance of semen can guide us: if it is clear, liquid and thin it indicates a condition of Deficiency, if thickened and yellow it indicates the presence of Heat or a condition of Excess.

In general, however, it is possible to perform a general treatment with acupuncture simply to invigorate the Kidney and promote male fertility [3] The treatment should be performed for at least 10 weeks, with weekly or bi-weekly sessions, in order to treat the man during an entire cycle of spermatogenesis. The main points, to be used in all subjects, are as follows:

CV4 (Guanyuan): the needle is inserted into the man with an empty bladder, the tip pointing downwards, to direct the deqi to the genitalia.

BL32 (Ciliao) is a very important local point, it should be needled preferably with a deep puncture (1.5–2 cun) penetrating into the sacral foramen; the deqi must reach the abdomen, perineum and genitals.

BL35 (Huiyang) is a point that is only used for infertility and coccygeal pain; the depth of insertion of the needle should be 3 cun, and the deqi must reach the perineum and genitals.

ST30 (Qichong) is a Yang Ming and Chong Mai point; if it is used for testicular problems the deqi should reach the testes, inserting the needle in the median and lower direction.

SP6 (Sanyinjiao): the tip of the needle points upwards.

A general treatment may include treatment with Chinese Pharmacology. According to Xu Fu-Song (1996), from the Nanjing University of TCM, quoted by Noll and Wilms (2009), the basic formula for all male problems is:

Bei Tu Tang (Dioscorea and Cuscuta Decoction)

Bei Xie	15g	(Rhizoma Dioscoreae Hypoglaucae)
Tu Si Zi	10g	(Semen Cuscutae Chinensis)
Fu Ling	15g	(Poria Cocos)
Che Qian Zi	9g	(Semen Plantaginis)
Ze Xie	9g	(Rhizoma Alismatis)
Mu Li	15g	(Ostreae Concha)
Gou Qi Zi	12g	(Fructus Lycii)
Xu Duan	12g	(Radix Dipsaci Asperi)
Shan Yao	20g	(Radix Dioscoreae Oppositae)
Sha Yuan Ji Li	20g	(Semen Astragali Complanati)
Dan Shen	20g	(Radix Salviae Miltiorrhizae)
Shi Chang Pu	3g	(Rhizome Acori Tatarinowii)
Huang Bai	12g	(Cortex Phellodendri)
Gan Cao	3g	(Radix Glycyrrhizae Uralensis)

The formula was created for all "male problems" such as impotence, spermatorrhea, bloody semen, low liquefaction, or chronic prostatitis [4, 5]. It can be changed according to the presentation of the subject. For example, if there is varicocele then herbs that move the Blood can be added, in Yang deficiency *Huang Bai* can be removed, *etc.*

CONSENT FOR PUBLICATION

Not applicable.

CONFLICT OF INTEREST

The author (editor) declares no conflict of interest, financial or otherwise.

ACKNOWLEDGEMENT

Declared none.

FURTHER READING

Chen ZQ, Li LY. Male & female infertility. Beijing: People's Medical Publishing House 2008.

Damone M. Principles of Chinese medical andrology: An Integrated Approach to Male Reproductive & Urological Health. Boulder, CO: Blue Poppy Press 2008.

Deadman P, Al-Khafaji M, Baker K. Manuale di agopuntura. Milano: Casa Editrice Ambrosiana 2000.

Di Stanislao C. Le metafore del corpo. Milano: CEA 2004.

Lewis R. The Infertility Cure. Boston, MA: Little, Brown and Co 2004.

Lyttleton J. Treatment of Infertility with Chinese Medicine. London: Churchill Livingstone 2013.

BIBLIOGRAPHY

[1]   Noll A, Wilms S. Chinese Medicine in Fertility Disorders. New York City, NY: Thieme 2009.

[2]   Xie Z. Best of Traditional Chinese Medicine. Beijing: New World Press 1995.

[3]   Deadman P. Seminar on male infertility Atti convegno della Società Italiana di Agopuntura. Milano 2008.

[4]   Xu F-S. J Chin Med 1996; 9(37): 532.

[5]   Noll A, Wilms S. Chinese Medicine in Fertility Disorders. New York City, NY: Thieme 2009.

CHAPTER 7

Classical Chinese Medicine in Male Infertility

Abstract: In Classical Chinese Medicine (CCM) the Kidney and Jing are at the root of reproduction. In CCM, the Kidney Jing is also nourished by the Jin Ye Fluids, which are lowered from the Lung. The Organs that have the most important role in male reproduction in CCM, in addition to the Kidney, are the Lung, the Spleen, and the Stomach. The formation of the Jin Ye Fluids and the points which control the formation of sperm are clearly described and discussed.

Keywords: Bao, Classical Chinese Medicine, Extraordinary Bowels, Fluids, Gallbladder, Gao, Jeffrey Yuen, Jin Fluids, Jin Ye, Jing, Jing-Ye, Ling Shu, Lung, Marrow, Kidney, Qi, Stomach, Su Wen, Turbid, Ye Fluids.

Both in Traditional Chinese Medicine (TCM) and Classical Chinese Medicine (CCM) the Kidney and Jing are at the root of the reproduction. In TCM the Spleen (postnatal Jing) helped by the Liver nourishes the Kidney Jing, and the Heart with its Ministerial Fire warms the water of the Kidney and of the Ming Men. In CCM, as taught by Jeffrey Yuen in his lectures in Italy, which have been systematized by Dr. Dante De Berardinis, the Kidney Jing is also nourished by the Jin Ye Fluids, which are lowered from the Lung. The Organs that have the most important role in male reproduction in CCM, in addition to the Kidney, are the Lung, the Spleen, and the Stomach.

The Kidney involved in reproduction is the Kidney Yin, because, unlike the Kidney Yang, it stores Jing. According to Van Nghi (comment to *Ling Shu* chap. 10), the Kidney collects and stores the excess Jing of all five Organs, then concentrates all the Jing of the body (anatomy, sexual, sensorial and mental/psychological Jing). The Jing kept in Kidney Yin is of two types: innate and acquired. The innate Jing corresponds to the matter with which we are born; it is a Yin substance of the Earlier Heaven inherited from our parents, and the basis of our constitution. It is the project that guides and directs the apposition of other matter, the acquired Jing, which is the essence of the food extracted by the Spleen. The Spleen transforms food and beverages, and from the five flavours it extracts the five Jing of the foods that are distributed to Organs and Bowels for storage.

The Jing is preserved also in the Extraordinary Bowels (*Ling Shu* chap. 10), which, according to Jeffrey Yuen, are an extension of the Kidney Yin.

The most important Extraordinary Bowels are two, the Marrow and the Bao. The other Extraordinary Bowels have functions of deposit (the Brain is the sea of Marrow, the Bones contain Marrow), nourishment (the Vessels nourish the Marrow and the Bao with Blood), and purification from Damp-Heat (*via* the Gall Bladder). As there are basically only two Extraordinary Bowels, so there are basically two types of Jing in the Extraordinary Bowels, the Jing-Marrow and the Jing-Seed, which are located respectively in the Marrow and in the Bao. The second is controlled by the "Jade" points and is related to male and female fertility. In women the Jing-Seed is associated with Blood Xue to form the oocyte (oocyte = Jing-Xue), while in men it is associated with Ye Fluids to form sperm (sperm = Jing-Ye). So the male Jing-Seed is the result of the union between innate Jing and acquired Jing, while Ye is the dense fraction of the Jin Ye Fluids. The Ye Fluids do not circulate in the meridians but are involved in all hormonal functions and can also be used to treat endocrinological problems.

The Lung has a key role in the formation of sperm. Zhang Shi, in his commentary on Chapter 4 of the *Ling Shu*, states that "the Lung is the source of the production of body fluids". When the Lung is unable to move the Ye Fluids down, male infertility develops due to secondary Kidney Yin deficiency. This would explain the presence of Kidney Yin deficiency as a cause of infertility in young men, who, one would expect, should still have a flourishing Yin. There are some features that suggest the involvement of the Lung in an infertile male. From a constitutional point of view, the man tends to be slender, pale. He typically has a great sense of justice: in front of an injustice he can never be indifferent, but reacts viscerally. He does not get angry but if triggered the violence may be out of control. In contrast to the anger of the Liver, which "barks and does not bite," the anger of the Lung is violent, smashing things *etc.*, up to total loss of control. He is generally more tired in the morning, may smoke, and usually prefers to drink sparkling water. Both cigarette smoke and sparkling water are in relation to the spicy flavour, which nourishes the Lung.

According to CCM the nutrition of the Bao occurs through different routes, which are described below.

NOURISHMENT OF THE BAO WITH QI

The relationship between Jing and the Ye Fluids is complex. Ye Fluids are the thick part of the Jin Ye Fluids (津液), which represent all the physiological fluids of the human body. Jin Fluids are thin, clear and watery and run with ease. They are distributed to the body surface (to the muscles, skin, and the orifices) and follow the movement of Qi and Blood facilitating their flow. The *Ling Shu* chap. 36 states *"[what accompanies] the clear Qi that emerges from the San Jiao to warm the muscles and flesh and infuse the skin, that is the Jin Fluid"*. Ye Fluids are distributed to Organs and Bowels, bones and joints, and to the brain and marrow. They do not flow with Qi and Blood because they are thick, viscous, and move slowly. Instead they can be considered as lubricants and moisturizers of the Jing. The *Ling Shu* chap. 36 states, *"[what] flows without moving, that's the Ye Fluid"* ... *"it gathers in the interior in very specific places without spreading to the exterior and has the name Ye Fluid"* and *"Jin Ye Fluids from the Five Grains can be combined harmoniously and form a thick substance that can percolate in the spaces of Bones and nourish and strengthen the Brain and Marrow"*.

Jin Ye Fluids are formed after a complex process of transformation and purification of the liquids ingested, with repeated separations of the turbid (Zhuo) from the clear (Qing), and a progressive refinement on one side and reuse of waste on the other side.

The process of formation of the Jin Ye Fluids starts from the Stomach. The *Su Wen* cap. 21 states: *"when the liquids enter the Stomach, its warming and steaming action carries the essential Qi to the Spleen. The Spleen then transports this Qi back up to the Lungs, where the Fluid pathway start to be regulated: the liquids are transported down the Bladder. The essential Qi of the Fluids is distributed to the four directions, reaching the skin and pouring into the channels of the 5 Organs. This is consistent with the nature of the four seasons and of the Yin and Yang of the 5 Organs, and it is part of the normal activities of the channels (Jing Mai)."*

The foods and liquids we ingest have a material part and an energetic part. The Stomach receives these foods and liquids and starts to warm them, separating the turbid from the clear. This process is controlled by the point **CV13** (Shangwan) (see Appendix 3). The turbid part, which corresponds to the material part without Qi, descends and is ejected through the pylorus into the Small Intestine (this process is under the control of the point **ST43** Xiangu). The Spleen completes the transformation and extraction of the essence Jing. In fact, as the *Su Wen* in the cap. 45 states: *"The Spleen helps the Stomach to move its Jin Ye Fluids."* A clear essence is then produced (*via* the point **ST45** Lidui) which rises to the Lung driven by the Spleen (helped by the point **SP18** Tianxi) to become Jin Fluids. In these actions, the Spleen is also helped by the Kidney Yang, the Ministerial Fire which controls the transformation and upwards transportation. Zhang Shi commenting on the *Ling Shu* chap. 1 states: *"the energy of the cereals penetrates into the Stomach and turns into Jing (pure energy, essence) that rises to the Lungs with the help of the Spleen; this energy of the cereals also turns into "Zhuoqi"* *(impure energy) that is collected at the level of the Intestines.*"

The turbid part of the liquids that enters the Small Intestine still contains a small part of Qi, so a second choice is made controlled by the point **CV11** (Jianli). The clear part, *via* the point **SI1** (Shaoze), is brought to the Kidney, from where it goes up to the Spleen and then to the Lung (*via* the point **SP6** Sanyinjiao), where it will be transformed into Ye Fluids. From the Small Intestine the turbid solid residual passes into the Large Intestine for the final extraction of Fluids, and the turbid liquid residual is transported by the Triple Burner to the Bladder. Li Dong Yuan in the Pi Wei Lun states: "*the Large Intestine regulates the Jin Fluids, the Small Intestine regulates the Ye Fluids* ".

Alterations of the first choice of the Stomach and of the second choice of the Small Intestine may manifest themselves with symptoms such as water retention in the stomach and dryness in the mouth, nose and skin without thirst, logorrhea and inability to choose between what is needed and what is not needed.

On their journey up to the Lungs, the Fluids must pass through the diaphragm Ge, where the pure part of the liquids extracted from the Stomach and the Small Intestine is separated into Jin Fluids and Ye Fluids. The diaphragm Ge represents a very important passage, which if blocked stops any type of process in the periphery. One possible cause of diaphragm blockage is the presence of Damp-Heat, which sidetracks the fluids going to the Lung and sends them instead to the mouth, causing the characteristic symptom of bitter mouth in the morning. The point used to purify Damp-Heat in the diaphragm is **GB38** (Yangfu). Other symptoms of blockage of the diaphragm can be heartburn and/or hiccups (treatable with **BL17** Geshu, **BL46** Geguan and **CV17** Danzhong), anxiety and panic attacks (**GV9** Zhiyang), dyspepsia (**LR10** Wuli), anger (**LR10** Zuwuli), gynecological problems such as ovarian cysts or uterine fibroids (**LR5** Ligou). These points are to be needled as well, only if tender on palpation.

At the Lung level, the Jin Ye Fluids are subjected to further processing, and subdivided into clear and turbid Jin, and clear and turbid Ye. The Lung distributes the Jin Fluids to the orifices, skin and Brain, while the Ye Fluids, which have a tendency to percolate and go inward, are sent down to the Kidney Yin.

At the Lung level the acquired Jing is produced. From the food and liquids arriving at the Stomach, the Spleen extracts the pure part (Jing) which rises as Guqi to the Lung, thanks to the ascending function of the Spleen. This step is controlled by the point **SP6** and, according to Jeffrey Yuen, also by all the points that have in their name the ideogram "Gu" 骨 (**LI4** Hegu, **LI16** Jugu, **SI4** Wangu, **CV2** Qugu, **KI10** Yingu, **GB8** Shuaigu, *etc.*). The Guqi goes through the diaphragm and reaches the chest where it is infused with the Heavenly Qi (Tian

Qi) creating the Zong Qi, or energy of the chest, while the turbid Qi is expelled in the expiration. The Zong Qi accumulates in the chest and provides the energy for respiration and for the movement of Qi and Blood through the channels (Jing Mai). Energized by Yuan Qi it becomes Zheng Qi (correct energy), which has two forms, Ying Qi and Wei Qi, and circulates both inside and outside of the channels as acquired Jing. Van Nghi in his commentary on the *Ling Shu* chap. 15 states: "*The Ying energy and the Wei energy have the same origin, they come from Jing (essence) of food. The Jing of food has two components: the "pure" component is the energy Ying, the "impure" component is the energy Wei. The terms "pure" and "impure" must not be taken literally, but denote the Yin and Yang nature of these essences.*"

In the chest the acquired Jing joins the clear and turbid Ye Fluids, forming the Gao. The Gao corresponds to the adipose tissue of Western medicine, in particular the brown fat, and has the function to nourish the Extraordinary Bowels and so the innate Jing (Jeffrey Yuen). The ideogram Gao 膏means fertile, watering, lubrification. In the Chinese tradition fats derive from essences extracted from the five flavours. The *Ling Shu* in chapter 36 states: "*the Jin Ye Fluids originating from the five grains (Wu Gu) can be transformed into Gao. In the interior the Gao permeates into the bony cavities and maintains the Marrows and the Brain, then it flows out toward the bottom, into the internal part of the thigh.*" Zhang Jie Bin in his commentary states that "*Jing Fluids and Ye Fluids harmoniously combined create the Gao that fills the void within the bones, it creates: the Brain, the Marrow, the Jing (Seed), the Blood.*"

The Gao is produced in the chest and is deposited between the heart and the diaphragm. This process is controlled by the point **BL43** (Gaohuangshu). The term "Gaohuang" can be translated as "vital region", while "Gaohuangshu" means "point to carry the Gao to nourish". The point **BL43**, which is on the side of the Back-shu point of the Pericardium, is traditionally used (because of its ability to access the Gao), to treat chronic diseases that penetrate at the level of Jing, usually considered incurable. Sun Simiao, with respect to the point **BL43**, states "there is no disease that cannot be treated" (*Prescriptions worth a thousand pieces of gold for every emergency*). In the classical texts, **BL43** is treated with moxibustion because needles are contraindicated.

From **BL43** the Gao is moved down to Dai Mai at the level of the navel (**KI16** Huangshu, to transport nutrition). **KI16** allows the Large Intestine to grasp the turbid Ye Fluids to eliminate Phlegm, and to grasp the Gao to nourish the Marrow through the Dai Mai. The Dai Mai in its function of nurturing and consolidation brings the Gao to **BL23** (Shenshu), in the posterior part of the body, passing through **BL52** (Zhishi). **BL23** is considered the origin of the Dai Mai according to the *Ling Shu* chap. 11: "*the Shao Yin meridian of the foot (...) reaches the Kidney and reconnects at the fourteenth vertebra to join with the Dai Mai*". The fourteenth vertebra (**L2**) is the area of Ming Men (**GV4**) and Shenyu (**BL23**), so the Dai Mai is anchored to the Ming Men and is connected to the energy of the Kidneys. From **BL52** one part of Gao goes up *via*BL51 (Huang Men, Gate of Huang) to go to the Jing-Marrow and the Brain, while another part goes down *via*BL53 (Baohuang, nutrition of the Bao) to nourish the Jing-Seed. The bifurcation of this pathway, where the Jing can go to the Brain or the Bao, it is the foundation of the Taoist sexual practices of ejaculation control. In fact, by avoiding the loss of Jing-seed, this could be transported as Jing-Marrow to nourish the Brain.

The points to activate this pathway of the Gao are **BL43** (Gaohuangshu) with needle and moxa, **BL53** (Baohuang), and **KI16** (Huangshu). All these points contain the ideogram Huang in their name (Huang = diaphragm, permeability). This combination seems more effective for male infertility with asthenozoospermia. Another point that can be added is **GB41** (Zulinqi), the opening point of Dai Mai, if there are symptoms of the Dai Mai (frequent sprains of the ankle, warm hands and cold feet, constipation, irritability), or if tender.

Another pathway of nutrition of the Jing-Ye sperm involves the descent of the turbid Ye Fluids.

According to the Imperial Academy of the Song era, the Lung moves energies and substances down, helped by the point **LU5** (Chize). The Ye Fluids are lowered from the Lung to the Kidney to nourish the Extraordinary Bowels, and in particular the Bao, by the point **LI16** (Jugu), which according to Van Nghi is the upper Sea of Marrow. The Stomach intervenes with its function to push down and facilitate the passage of Fluids from the Lung to the Kidney. The point **ST36** (Zusanli) is used in TCM because stimulating the lowering function is critical to the success of the treatment. The Kidney grabs the Ye Fluids pushed down by the Lung through the point **KI11** (Henggu) (secondary name Suikong, empty Marrow). If there are problems at this level, the symptoms reported by the patients will be referred to the stagnation of turbid Ye Fluids in the Bladder (Lin syndrome) and in the Large Intestine (diarrhea), while the Marrows will be empty. Through this point the turbid Ye Fluids go from the Kidney to the Gao, which as we have seen nourishes the Extraordinary Bowels and the Jing-Seed. The points to activate this pathway are **LI16** (Jugu), **ST36** (Zusanli) and **KI11** (Henggu). This combination seems more effective for male infertility with oligozoospermia.

The nourishment of the Bao involves movements of ascent and descent between the Upper and Lower Burner that are mediated by the Middle Burner (Stomach for the descent, and Spleen the ascent). A blockage at some level will favour the formation of Phlegm (stagnating above) or Dampness (stagnating at the bottom), which block the formation and nutrition of Jing.

This can happen because of an alteration of the lowering function of the Lung (controlled by **LI16** Jugu), or an alteration of the descending function of the Stomach (controlled by **ST36** Zusanli or from other points of the Meridian Yangming), or an alteration of the Fluid grasping function by the Kidney (controlled by the points between **KI11** and **KI16**). The Phlegm that does not descend can then head upwards and give trouble to the orifices.

When the mechanisms of ascent are altered, Dampness forms below. For CCM this is due to a defective ascending function of the Spleen (this function is controlled by **SP9** Yinlingquan). Dampness can also originate from a defective Lower Burner function (by Large Intestine and Bladder) of eliminating impure liquids, or from a defective Dai Mai function which fails to eliminate Dampness. The two functions of the Dai Mai, consolidation and Dampness elimination, are represented by the two trajectories of the Dai Mai described in the classics. The trajectory described in the Da Cheng, which starts from **BL23** (Shenshu) goes to **GB26** (Daimai), **ST25** (Tianshu) and **KI16** (Huangshu) and ends at **CV8** (Shenque), corresponds to the consolidating function, *i.e.* nourishes Jing. Symptoms of the blocking of ascent by this route include hemorrhoids, anal fissures, fistulae, sacrococcigeal cysts *etc*. Treatment consists of needling **GB41** (Zulinqi), **GB26** (Daimai) and **KI16** (Huangshu). The trajectory starting from **LR13** (Zhangmen) and going to **GB26** (Daimai), **GB27** (Wushu), and **GB28** (Weidao) corresponds to the function of elimination of Dampness and of anything that stagnates. This trajectory has been described by Li Shizhen: "*Dai Mai originates from the point Zhangmen (**LR13**) on the Jue Yin meridian of the foot, at the level of the last ribs. Together with the Shao Yang of the foot it runs along the Daimai point (**GB26**). It makes a complete circular tour of the body, like a tied belt. It meets again the Shao Yang Foot at Wushu (**GB27**) and Weidao (**GB28**). A total of eight points.*"

In this perspective it is possible to recognize the syndromes of Dampness due to deficiency or excess described by TCM. The first syndrome is caused by a deficiency of Spleen Qi causing the stagnation of Fluids in the Lower Burner; the point to be treated is **CV4** (Guanyuan). The syndrome of Dampness due to excess is determined by a vicious cycle in which an alteration in the Lower Burner or in the Dai Mai results in the accumulation of Dampness which blocks the ascending function of the Spleen, which creates more Dampness. The points to be treated are **CV2** (Qugu) or **CV6** (Qihai), with moxa.

NOURISHMENT OF THE BAO WITH QI

The role of the Lung in fertility is mediated not only by the Fluids, but also by Lung Qi and Blood.

In addition to moving the Fluids, the Lung also moves Qi throughout the body. The classics state that, with each inhalation and exhalation, Qi moves three cun along the meridians (*Ling Shu* chap. 15). So the breath, in other words the Lung, moves Qi by lowering Tian Qi and so allowing Qi to reach the Lower Burner, in order to give "oxygen" to the fire which corresponds to Yuan Qi. For this reason, in Lung Qi deficiency the first symptom is fatigue; the Lung does not allow Tian Qi to reach the Lower Burner and therefore Qi is not produced. This kind of fatigue typically occurs in the morning.

The point **BL10** (Tianzhu) allows the breath to reach the Lower Burner. The alteration of this mechanism is the basis of frigidity and impotence, as well as infertility.

NOURISHMENT OF THE BAO WITH BLOOD

The Lung also contributes to the process of fertility with its Blood. Blood is the residence of the Shen, and the Lung Shen is the Po. The Po is connected to all our automatic responses that promote life, it maintains the body's rhythms, metabolism and homeostasis, and it also regulates the entry and the exit into life and into death, as the beginning and end of all the events, with its close connection with the Jing. As the *Ling Shu* chap. 8 states: "*the origin of life is Jing. The spirit that bears the Jing is called Po.*" While the Hun comes from a Yang Organ, the Liver, and it follows the Jing of Fire (Shen), the Po comes from a Yin organ, the Lung, and so it follows the Jing of Water (Jing) which is a Yin substance. For this reason the Po has a key role in procreation: the Po, together with the Shen from Heaven (Hun), descends into the fertilized oocyte, resulting from the union of the Jing of the parents, and allows the embodiment of the new being, and the passage from non-form to form.

The point to bring down the Po is **LI14** (Binao) in moxa. In the treatment of infertility sine causa, in addition to **LI14**, it is possible to also use **ST36** (Zusanli) to help the descent and **KI13** (Qixue) to help the Bao grab the Po.

To nourish the Jing-seed *via* the Blood it is also possible to use the Liao points (**BL31** Shangliao, **BL32** Ciliao, **BL33** Zhongliao, and **BL34** Xialiao). Liao points, located at the sacral level, correspond to the Huatuo points, which distribute Weiqi at the spine level and nourish the Jing-Marrow *via* the Blood. At the pelvic level the Liao points do not nourish the Jing-Marrow but the Jing-seed *via* the

Blood. The most used Liao point in TCM is **BL32** (Ciliao), which in CCM has the function of stimulating the passage of Gao to the Extraordinary Bowels, Uterus and Bone.

In this approach the needles are inserted to a depth of 0.5–1 cun, and left in place for 28 minutes. The choice of this length of time is based on the *Ling Shu*. In the 15th chapter it states that Qi and Blood perform a complete round through all the meridians in two units of time, while in the 18th chapter it is stated directly that Qi and Blood flow through the meridians 50 times a day. At the time when the *Ling Shu* was written a day was divided into 100 units of time, and both statements lead us to calculate that 28 minutes and 48 seconds is the time in which Qi and Blood make a full round in the meridians.

CONSENT FOR PUBLICATION

Not applicable.

CONFLICT OF INTEREST

The author (editor) declares no conflict of interest, financial or otherwise.

ACKNOWLEDGEMENT

Declared none.

FURTHER READING

Clavey S. Fluid Physiology and Pathology in Traditional Chinese Medicine. Amsterdam, Netherlands: Elsevier 2005.

De Berardinis D. Obesità e controllo della fame in agopuntura. Mosciano SA: ID'O Ed 2006.

De Berardinis D. Il Polmone - dalla fisiologia alla clinica. Edizioni SIDA.

Finestrali. Il concetto di "Jing" in Medicina Cinese Tradizionale, proposta di un nuovo modello interpretativo. Available from: http://webhtml.agopuntura.org/html/mandorla/rivista/numeri/Marzo_1999/jing.htm

Innocenzi P. Trattamento delle infertilità maschili in agopuntura. Tesi AMSA 2006–2007. Available from: http://www.agopuntura.org/wp-content/uploads/2015/05/Infertilita_maschile_Paola_Innocenzi_2006_2007.pdf

Unschuld PU, Tessenow H. Huang Di Nei Jing Su Wen. An Annotated Translation of Huang Di's Inner Classic – Basic Questions: 2 volumes, Volumes of the Huang Di Nei Jing Su Wen Project. Oakland, CA: University of California Press 2011.

Van Nghi N, Viet Dzung T, Recours Nguyen C. Huangdi Neijing Lingshu. NVN Edition. Sugar Grove, NC: Jung Tao School of Classical Chinese Medicine 2002.

CHAPTER 8

Clinical and Experimental Studies of Acupuncture in Male Infertility

Abstract: The published scientific studies on acupuncture in male infertility are reviewed in this chapter. In general, they are of poor quality in both the study design and the low number of patients treated, but some studies suggest a role for acupuncture in male infertility.

Keywords: Acupoint, Autonomic Nervous System, Baseline, Blind, Control, Controlled, Diffuse Noxious Inhibitory Control, DNIC, Double Blind, Nerve Fiber, Neuroendocrine, Neurotrophin, Opioid peptide, Placebo, Prospective, Protocol, Reticular Formation, Review, Randomized, Treatment.

ACUPUNCTURE IN MALE INFERTILITY

There are few studies in English on the use of acupuncture in male infertility. In general, they are of poor quality in both the study design and the low number of patients treated, but some studies suggest a role for acupuncture in male infertility.

We summarize here the main papers on the subject.

Jiasheng (1987) reported that 74% of 248 cases of male infertility responded to a 20-day treatment with acupuncture [1]. Subjects were classified into five different diagnostic categories according to the principles of TCM. The deficiency syndromes were Yang deficiency, Yin deficiency, stagnation of Liver Qi, or Damp-Heat. The points treated in all subjects were **BL23** (Shenshu), **BL32** (Ciliao), **CV4** (Guanyuan) and **ST30** (Qichong). These other points were added depending on the clinical picture: **ST36** (Zusanli), **KI3** (Taixi), **SP6** (Sanyinjiao), **LR3** (Taichong), **GV4** (Mingmen) and **FM12** (Huatuojiaji). In subjects with Yang deficiency moxibustion was applied on **CV4** (Guanyuan) for 20 minutes.

A prospective study was conducted on 16 subjects who could not conceive for an average of five years [2]. Most of the subjects had teratozoospermia (44%) and asthenozoospermia (25%), the others had oligozoospermia, astheno-teratozoospermia, oligoteratozoospermia and OTA syndrome. All subjects showed semen bacterial contamination. The acupuncture treatment consisted of 10 sessions for five weeks. The points treated, with achievement of Deqi, were **LU7** (Lieque), **LI4** (Hegu), **LI11** (Quchi), **ST36** (Zusanli), **ST30** (Qichong), **SP6** (Sanyinjiao), **SP9** (Yinlingguan), **SP10** (Xuehai), **HT7** (Shenmen), **BL20** (Pishu), **BL23** (Shenshu), **BL33** (Zhongliao), **KI6** (Zhaohai), **KI7** (Fuliu), **PC6** (Neiguan), **LR5** (Ligou), **LR8** (Quguan), **CV1** (Huiyin), **CV2** (Qugu), **CV4** (Guanyuan), **CV6** (Qihai), **GV4** (Mingmen). Based on the diagnosis according to the principles of TCM, the above points were chosen in specific combinations which have not been described in the text. Semen analysis was performed at baseline and at one month after the end of treatment with acupuncture. Sperm viability and the total count of motile sperm significantly improved after treatment with acupuncture (from 52% to 65% and from 8.5 million to 19.3 million, respectively). The evaluation with electron microscopy showed a significant increase in the percentage of sperm with intact axoneme (from 32% to 51%), probably due to a reduction of lipid peroxidation of sperm.

A subsequent study examined 20 subjects with azoospermia [3]. The acupuncture treatment consisted of 10 sessions twice weekly for five weeks. Subjects were subdivided into two broad traditional diagnostic syndromes, "Kidney deficiency" (corresponding to spermatogenic failure) and "Damp-Heat in the genital system" (corresponding to inflammation of the genital tract). The main acupoints for both syndromes were **SP6** (Sanyinjiao), **CV4** (Guanyuan), **LU7** (Lieque), **KI6** (Zhaohai) and **ST30** (Qichong). If Kidney Yang deficiency was present, four other main acupoints were used: **KI3** (Taixi), **KI11** (Henggu), **BL23** (Shenshu) and **BL52** (Zhishi). If Damp-Heat was present, another five main acupoints were used: **SP9** (Yinlingguan), **LR5** (Ligou), **LR11** (Quchi), **ST28** (Shuidao) and **GB41** (Zuliqi). Other acupoints unrelated to the previous diagnoses were considered as secondary acupoints: **LI4** (Hegu), **ST36** (Zusanli), **SP10** (Xuehai), **HT7** (Shenmen), **BL20** (Pishu), **PC6** (Neiguan), **CV1** (Huiyin), **CV2** (Qugu), **CV6** (Qihai), **GV4** (Mingmen), **GV20** (Baihui), **GB20** (Fengchi), **GB27** (Wushu), **LR3** (Taichong) and **KI7** (Fuliu). For each subject a combination of primary and secondary acupoints was selected, with up to 12 acupoints in total. One month after the end of treatment with acupuncture, a significant improvement of sperm production was found, particularly in patients with inflammation of the genital tract, without modification of the other biochemical and cytological parameters. Two subjects attempted ICSI, obtaining two pregnancies, one of which ended with a miscarriage.

Gurfinkel *et al.* (2003) evaluated 19 subjects with seminal abnormalities but without azoospermia and leukocytospermia in a prospective, controlled, randomized and blinded study [4]. The subjects were randomized into two groups. The first group received a treatment in classical acupoints: **ST30** (Qichong), **ST36**

(Zusanli), **SP4** (Gongsun), **SP6** (Sanyinjiao), **LR3** (Taichong), **KI3** (Taixi), **LI4** (Hegu) and **PC6** (Neiguan), and a treatment with moxa in the following points: **BL13** (Feishu), **BL14** (Jueyinshu), **BL15** (Xinshu), **BL20** (Pishu), **BL21** (Weishu), **BL22** (Sanjiaoshu), **BL23** (Shenshu), **BL32** (Ciliao), **BL52** (Zhishi), **CV3** (Zhongji), **CV4** (Guanyuan), **CV5** (Shimen), **CV6** (Qihai), **GV4** (Mingmen), **LU9** (Taiyuan), **LR14** (Qimen) and **Zigong** (4 cun below the navel and 3 cun laterally to **CV3**). The second group received a treatment at indifferent acupoints located centrally, on the anterior superior iliac spines and in the acromioclavicular regions, and a treatment with moxa dorsally, on the shoulder blade and the posterior inferior spine. Treatment was twice weekly for 10 weeks. The analysis of the sperm after the end of treatment showed a significant increase in the percentage of sperm with normal morphology, while the volume, concentration and progressive motility were not statistically different.

Zhang *et al.* (2003) studied 22 patients with idiopathic infertility who had failed an attempt at ICSI [5]. The acupuncture treatment consisted of 10 sessions for five weeks. The following acupoints were treated: **GV20** (Baihui), **PC6** (Neiguan), **LU5** (Chize), **SP10** (Xuehai), **ST44** (Neiting), **BL23** (Shenshu) and **SP6** (Sanyinjiao). Within three months after the end of treatment subjects had their sperm analysed and underwent ICSI. Sperm motility and the percentage of normal sperm were significantly increased after acupuncture. The fertility rate after acupuncture was 66%, significantly greater than the pre-acupuncture rate.

Lun and Rong (2003) studied 100 men with infertility for at least two years and with positive antisperm antibodies [6]. According to TCM theory, the clinical manifestations of infertility due to hypofunction of the immune system or a lack of immunosuppressive factors are attributable to a weak body resistance, while the production of antisperm antibodies generated by inflammation, trauma or obstruction belong to the category of excess of pathogenic factors. Thus a disease could be attributed to a deficiency of resistance, or an excess of pathogenic factors, or a mixed syndrome of deficiency and excess. The root causes of infertility are Liver and Kidney deficiency, while the outside manifestations are those of Qi and Blood stagnation, so treatment is aimed to strengthen the body and eliminate the pathogenic Factors. The pairs of points **BL18** (Ganshu) combined with **LR3** (Taichong), and **BL23** (Shenshu) combined with **KI3** (Taixi), can strengthen both the Liver and the Kidney, leading to strengthening and stabilization of the body and of its immune function. **BL15** (Xinshu) is combined with **HT7** (Shenmen) because the Heart dominates the vessels, and if the Qi of the Heart is full, then Qi and Blood can circulate normally. **BL17** (Geshu) combined with **SP10** (Xuehai) can promote Blood circulation to remove Blood stasis, improve blood circulation, reduce ischemic and hypoxic states, improve cell metabolism and speed up cellular healing. **BL22** (Sanjiaoshu) combined with **TE4** (Yangchi) can eliminate the Heat, toxic materials and pathogens, eliminate Heat and Dampness from the Lower Burner, remove inflammatory metabolic products, suppress the growth of germs and create the conditions for the regeneration of tissues.

Subjects were randomized to a group treated with electroacupuncture (EA) and a group treated with prednisone 5 mg three times a day for eight weeks. EA treatment consisted of five sessions per week for eight weeks. The points were **BL15** (Xinshu), **BL17** (Geshu), **BL18** (Ganshu), **BL22** (Sanjiaoshu), **BL23** (Shenshu), **LR3** (Taichong), **KI3** (Taixi), **HT7** (Shenmen), **TE4** (Yangchi) and **SP10** (Xuehai). After the onset of Deqi the needles were manipulated with a frequency of 180–200 turns/min for 5 min, then were left for 10 min and the manipulation was repeated for another 5 min. Then the needles were stimulated with EA, at a frequency of 14–26 Hz, for a duration of 30 min. The outcomes were the pregnancy of the partners and the negativity of antisperm antibodies for three months. 40% of patients undergoing EA responded favourably compared to 10% of subjects treated with prednisone.

Pei *et al.* (2005) evaluated the sperm ultrastructural characteristics of 40 men with idiopathic infertility and low sperm counts, asthenozoospermia or teratozoospermia in a prospective randomized controlled trial [7]. 28 men were treated with acupuncture two times a week for 10 weeks. The main acupoints used were: **CV4** (Guanyuan), **BL23** (Shenshu), **BL32** (Ciliao), **LR3** (Taichong) and **KI3** (Taixi), bilaterally. Secondary acupoints were: **ST36** (Zusanli), **SP10** (Xuehai), **SP6** (Sanyinjiao), **ST29** (Guilai) and **GV20** (Baihui). Deqi was sought. After the acupuncture treatment the sperm of treated subjects showed a statistically significant improvement in total motility, in the percentage and number of healthy sperm, in acrosomes in the normal position and of normal form, in the nuclear shape, in the form and pattern of axonemes, and in the accessory fibres.

Dieterle *et al.* (2009) in a prospective, randomized, single-blind, placebo-controlled study, compared 28 infertile men treated with acupuncture according to the principles of TCM with 29 infertile men treated with placebo acupuncture [8]. "True" acupuncture led to a significant increase in sperm motility, but not concentration, compared to the control group.

Siterman *et al.* (2009) studied 39 infertile men suffering from azoospermia (n = 35) or severe oligozoospermia (n = 4) [9]. 18 fertile patients represented the control for the threshold of the scrotal temperature. According to the established threshold of 30.5°C, at baseline 34 infertile men had an increased scrotal temperature, while 5 infertile men had a normal temperature. Infertile men were divided into two diagnostic categories, Kidney deficiency (corresponding to hormonal imbalance) or Damp-Heat syndrome (corresponding to inflammation of the genital tract). Treatment with acupuncture was performed in 8–10 sessions twice a week. The two syndromes were both treated with the following points: **SP6** (Sanyinjiao), **CV4** (Guanyuan), **LU7** (Lieque), **KI6** (Zhohai) and **ST30** (Qicong). For Kidney deficiency the following main points were added: **KI3** (Taixi), **BL23** (Shenshu), **KI11** (Henggu) and **BL52** (Zhishi), while for Damp-Heat the following main points were added: **SP9** (Yinlingqua n), **LR5** (Ligou), **LI11** (Quchi), **ST28** (Shuidao) and **GB41** (Zuliqi). For each patient, some secondary points were selected according to the criteria of traditional acupuncture, selected from the following: **LI4** (Hegu), **ST36** (Zusanli), **SP10** (Xuehai), **HT7** (Shenmen), **BL20** (Pishu), **PC6** (Neiguan), **CV1** (Huiyin), **CV2** (Qugu), **CV6** (Qihai), **GV4** (Mingmen), **GV20** (Baihui), **GB20** (Fengchi), **LR3** (Taichong), **KI7** (Fulu) and **GB27** (Wushu). No more than 12 acupoints were used in each session. At the end of treatment, 17 men with increased scrotal temperature and inflammation of the genital tract showed a drop in temperature and an improvement of semen analysis, while the other 17 men with increased scrotal temperature and the 5 men with normal scrotal temperature showed no change.

Rinaldi *et al.* (2012) examined seven men (age range 32–47) with abnormal spermiograms and failure of previous drug treatments [10]. Treatment was administered in cycles of four weeks with three sessions per week on alternate days, and consisted of the application of the following techniques: 1) acupuncture on **CV4** (Guanyuan) and **CV3** (Zhongji) in tonification; after obtaining deqi, the needles were maintained in situ for 20 minutes and stimulated every 5 min with a slow rotation, irradiating the deqi towards the testicles and/or to the perineum; 2) warm needle technique on **ST36** (Zusanli), **KI16** (Zhaohai) and **KI3** (Taixi); after obtaining deqi 2–3 pieces of moxa cigar were applied on the needles; 3) treatment of **CV1** (Huiyin) alternating direct moxibustion (three medium size cones of moxa) with Tuina treatment, using stable pressure with the tip of the middle finger held between thumb and forefinger (zhiyafa) together with various visualizations. After the first cycle four out of seven subjects showed improvement of semen analysis. Four men after the 2nd cycle, and one man after the 3rd cycle, were able to conceive naturally without ART.

POSSIBLE MECHANISMS OF ACTION OF ACUPUNCTURE

The increasing amount of studies on the mechanisms of acupuncture, which began in the 1980s, led to the discovery of the involvement of different systems relating to the nervous, vascular, immune and endocrine spheres.

Acupuncture consists in the stimulation of skin areas with different methods including the insertion of thin needles that can be manipulated manually or electrically. The acupoints, anatomically well-defined areas where needles traditionally pierce the skin to stimulate specific responses, are areas rich in sensitive nerve endings of small diameter and high threshold, which are able to generate action potentials that propagate through type A delta and C nerve fibres [11, 12]. At the level of the posterior column the stimulation can form a reflex arc or can ascend to the reticular formation, the thalamus and the grey matter.

From these structures a series of neural responses proceed, *via* the diffuse noxious inhibitory control (DNIC) to the convergent neurons at the medullary and spinal levels [13], *via* the autonomic nervous system [14, 15], and the descending inhibitory system [16], and *via* a series of humoral responses, both at the central and the peripheral level, with the release of endogenous opioid peptides (Met- and Leu-enkephalin, dynorphin) or stress hormones (CRF, ACTH, corticosterone), serotonin, *etc.* [17 - 21].

The opioid peptides in the periphery may have not only an analgesic role [22], but also effects on non-analgesic systems, such as the immune system, modulating allergic [23] and inflammatory processes [24, 25]. At the testicular level, animal and human studies suggest a role of opioid peptides in sperm motility and fertility [26, 27].

Other systems of mediators are involved in the modulation of the effects of acupuncture. Several neuropeptides have been reported such as substance P, neurokinin A, neuropeptide Y, VIP (Vasoactive Intestinal Peptide), bradykinin, CGRP (calcitonin gene-related peptide); various cytokines (IL-1b, IL-2, IL-4, IL-6, IL-10), IFN-g, TNF-a, and other substances such as nitric oxide and serotonin [28].

At the neuroendocrine level, acupuncture modulates various neurotrophins such as nerve growth factor (NGF), glial-derived neurotrophic factor (GDNF), brain-derived neurotrophic factor (BDNF) *etc.* [29]. NGF is a protein essential for the development and maintenance of sensory neurons of the peripheral nervous system [30]. NGF interacts with two distinct receptors: one was identified as the proto-oncogene product of the trk (generally designated as TrkA) and is a typical growth factor receptor. The second receptor, called LNGFR (low-affinity NGF receptor), does not have these characteristics [31].

NGF is an important mediator in the development of polycystic ovary syndrome (PCOS), the leading endocrine cause of female infertility [32], and is capable of modulating the response to acupuncture in infertile women with polycystic ovaries [33]. NGF may also play a role in male infertility, as NGF and its receptors have been detected in the testis of rodents and humans, where they could have a role in testicular morphogenesis and function [34]. A positive immunoreactivity for NGF was reported in the testis of adult mice and rats, where it appears localized in the germline cells. The human testis contains 5.44 ng of ß-NGF per g of weight [35]. NGF receptors in humans are localized at the level of the cells of the lamina propria. In rats they are present in the embryonic testis and at various stages of the seminiferous cycle. In addition, knock-out mice for the gene encoding the TrkA receptor are infertile when they manage to reach adulthood [36].

It is not known what the cellular and molecular effects of acupuncture are in the testicles. However, some acupuncture mediators like the opioids are present in the testis and in semen, where they seem to modulate sperm motility, and NGF may also play a role.

CONSENT FOR PUBLICATION

Not applicable.

CONFLICT OF INTEREST

The author (editor) declares no conflict of interest, financial or otherwise.

ACKNOWLEDGEMENT

Declare none.

FURTHER READING

Franconi G, Manni L, Aloe L, *et al*. Acupuncture in clinical and experimental reproductive medicine: a review. J Endocrinol Invest 2011; 34: 307–11.

Hansen M, Kurinczuk JJ, Bower C, *et al*. The risk of major birth defects after intracytoplasmic sperm injection and *in vitro* fertilization. NEJM 2002; 346(10): 725–30.

Seidl K, Holstein A-F. Organ culture of human seminiferous tubules: a useful tool to study the role of nerve growth factor in the testis. Cell Tissue Res 1990; 261: 539–47.

BIBLIOGRAPHY

[1]   Jiasheng Z. Male infertility treated with acupuncture and moxibustion: a report of 248 cases. Zhongguo Zhenjiu 1987; 7: 3-4.

[2]   Siterman S, Eltes F, Wolfson V, Zabludovsky N, Bartoov B. Effect of acupuncture on sperm parameters of males suffering from subfertility related to low sperm quality. Arch Androl 1997; 39(2): 155-61.

[http://dx.doi.org/10.3109/01485019708987914] [PMID: 9272232]

[3] Siterman S, Eltes F, Wolfson V, Lederman H, Bartoov B. Does acupuncture treatment affect sperm density in males with very low sperm count? A pilot study. Andrologia 2000; 32(1): 31-9.
[http://dx.doi.org/10.1111/j.1439-0272.2000.tb02862.x] [PMID: 10702864]

[4] Gurfinkel E, Cedenho AP, Yamamura Y, Srougi M. Effects of acupuncture and moxa treatment in patients with semen abnormalities. Asian J Androl 2003; 5(4): 345-8.
[PMID: 14695986]

[5] Zhang MM, Huang GY, Tan LX, *et al.* Treatment of idiopathic male infertility by acupuncture combined with intracytoplasmic injection of sperm. Acupunct Res 2003; 28: 147-50.

[6] Lun X, Rong L. Effect of electroacupuncture on antisperm antibodies in male infertility patients. World J Acupunct Moxibustion 2003; 13: 9-13.

[7] Pei J, Strehler E, Noss U, *et al.* Quantitative evaluation of spermatozoa ultrastructure after acupuncture treatment for idiopathic male infertility. Fertil Steril 2005; 84(1): 141-7.
[http://dx.doi.org/10.1016/j.fertnstert.2004.12.056] [PMID: 16009169]

[8] Dieterle S, Li C, Greb R, Bartzsch F, Hatzmann W, Huang D. A prospective randomized placebo-controlled study of the effect of acupuncture in infertile patients with severe oligoasthenozoospermia. Fertil Steril 2009; 92(4): 1340-3.
[http://dx.doi.org/10.1016/j.fertnstert.2009.02.041] [PMID: 19394002]

[9] Siterman S, Eltes F, Schechter L, Maimon Y, Lederman H, Bartoov B. Success of acupuncture treatment in patients with initially low sperm output is associated with a decrease in scrotal skin temperature. Asian J Androl 2009; 11(2): 200-8.
[http://dx.doi.org/10.1038/aja.2008.4] [PMID: 19122677]

[10] Rinaldi R, *et al.* Trattamento combinato con agomoxibustione e tuina-qigong di 7 casi affetti da infertilità maschile Orientamenti MTC 2012; 29: 18-25.

[11] Lu GW, Xie JQ, Yang J, Wang YN, Wang QL. Afferent nerve fiber composition at point Zusanli in relation to acupuncture analgesia. A functional morphologic investigation. Chin Med J (Engl) 1981; 94(4): 255-63.
[PMID: 6790242]

[12] Dornette WH. The anatomy of acupuncture. Bull N Y Acad Med 1975; 51(8): 895-902.
[PMID: 1058714]

[13] Bing Z, Villanueva L, Le Bars D. Acupuncture and diffuse noxious inhibitory controls: naloxone-reversible depression of activities of trigeminal convergent neurons. Neuroscience 1990; 37(3): 809-18.
[http://dx.doi.org/10.1016/0306-4522(90)90110-P] [PMID: 2247225]

[14] Nishijo K, Mori H, Yosikawa K, Yazawa K. Decreased heart rate by acupuncture stimulation in humans *via* facilitation of cardiac vagal activity and suppression of cardiac sympathetic nerve. Neurosci Lett 1997; 227(3): 165-8.
[http://dx.doi.org/10.1016/S0304-3940(97)00337-6] [PMID: 9185676]

[15] Stener-Victorin E, Lundeberg T, Cajander S, *et al.* Steroid-induced polycystic ovaries in rats: effect of electro-acupuncture on concentrations of endothelin-1 and nerve growth factor (NGF), and expression of NGF mRNA in the ovaries, the adrenal glands, and the central nervous system. Reprod Biol Endocrinol 2003; 1: 33.
[http://dx.doi.org/10.1186/1477-7827-1-33] [PMID: 12725645]

[16] Han JS, Terenius L. Neurochemical basis of acupuncture analgesia. Annu Rev Pharmacol Toxicol 1982; 22: 193-220.
[http://dx.doi.org/10.1146/annurev.pa.22.040182.001205] [PMID: 7044284]

[17] Bucinskaite V, Theodorsson E, Crumpton K, Stenfors C, Ekblom A, Lundeberg T. Effects of repeated sensory stimulation (electro-acupuncture) and physical exercise (running) on open-field behaviour and

concentrations of neuropeptides in the hippocampus in WKY and SHR rats. Eur J Neurosci 1996; 8(2): 382-7.
[http://dx.doi.org/10.1111/j.1460-9568.1996.tb01221.x] [PMID: 8714708]

[18]   Joos S, Schott C, Zou H, Daniel V, Martin E. Immunomodulatory effects of acupuncture in the treatment of allergic asthma: a randomized controlled study. J Altern Complement Med 2000; 6(6): 519-25.
[http://dx.doi.org/10.1089/acm.2000.6.519] [PMID: 11152056]

[19]   Mittleman E, Gaynor JS. A brief overview of the analgesic and immunologic effects of acupuncture in domestic animals. J Am Vet Med Assoc 2000; 217(8): 1201-5.
[http://dx.doi.org/10.2460/javma.2000.217.1201] [PMID: 11043693]

[20]   Stener-Victorin E, Lundeberg T, Waldestrom U, *et al.* Effects of electro-acupuncture on corticotrophin releasing-factor (CRF) in rats with experimentally induced polycystic ovaries. Neuropeptides 2002; 35: 1-5.

[21]   Li A, Zhang RX, Wang Y, *et al.* Corticosterone mediates electroacupuncture-produced anti-edema in a rat model of inflammation. BMC Complement Altern Med 2007; 7: 27.
[http://dx.doi.org/10.1186/1472-6882-7-27] [PMID: 17697336]

[22]   He LF. Involvement of endogenous opioid peptides in acupuncture analgesia. Pain 1987; 31(1): 99-121.
[http://dx.doi.org/10.1016/0304-3959(87)90011-X] [PMID: 3320881]

[23]   Kasahara T, Amemiya M, Wu Y, Oguchi K. Involvement of central opioidergic and nonopioidergic neuroendocrine systems in the suppressive effect of acupuncture on delayed type hypersensitivity in mice. Int J Immunopharmacol 1993; 15(4): 501-8.
[http://dx.doi.org/10.1016/0192-0561(93)90064-6] [PMID: 8365824]

[24]   Zijlstra FJ, van den Berg-de Lange I, Huygen FJPM, Klein J. Anti-inflammatory actions of acupuncture. Mediators Inflamm 2003; 12(2): 59-69.
[http://dx.doi.org/10.1080/0962935031000114943] [PMID: 12775355]

[25]   Kavoussi B, Ross BE. The neuroimmune basis of anti-inflammatory acupuncture. Integr Cancer Ther 2007; 6(3): 251-7.
[http://dx.doi.org/10.1177/1534735407305892] [PMID: 17761638]

[26]   O'Hara BF, Donovan DM, Lindberg I, *et al.* Proenkephalin transgenic mice: a short promoter confers high testis expression and reduced fertility. Mol Reprod Dev 1994; 38(3): 275-84.
[http://dx.doi.org/10.1002/mrd.1080380308] [PMID: 7917279]

[27]   El-Haggar S, El-Ashmawy S, Attia A, *et al.* Beta-endorphin in serum and seminal plasma in infertile men. Asian J Androl 2006; 8(6): 709-12.
[http://dx.doi.org/10.1111/j.1745-7262.2006.00180.x] [PMID: 16751995]

[28]   Zijlstra FJ, Van Den Berg-De Lange I, Huygen FJPM, *et al.* 2003.

[29]   Liang XB, Liu XY, Li FQ, *et al.* Long-term high-frequency electro-acupuncture stimulation prevents neuronal degeneration and up-regulates BDNF mRNA in the substantia nigra and ventral tegmental area following medial forebrain bundle axotomy. Brain Res Mol Brain Res 2002; 108(1-2): 51-9.
[http://dx.doi.org/10.1016/S0169-328X(02)00513-2] [PMID: 12480178]

[30]   Levi-Montalcini R. The nerve growth factor 35 years later. Science 1987; 237(4819): 1154-62.
[http://dx.doi.org/10.1126/science.3306916] [PMID: 3306916]

[31]   Gnessi L, Fabbri A, Spera G. Gonadal peptides as mediators of development and functional control of the testis: an integrated system with hormones and local environment. Endocr Rev 1997; 18(4): 541-609.
[PMID: 9267764]

[32]   Dissen GA, Garcia-Rudaz C, Paredes A, Mayer C, Mayerhofer A, Ojeda SR. Excessive ovarian production of nerve growth factor facilitates development of cystic ovarian morphology in mice and is

a feature of polycystic ovarian syndrome in humans. Endocrinology 2009; 150(6): 2906-14.
[http://dx.doi.org/10.1210/en.2008-1575] [PMID: 19264868]

[33] Stener-Victorin E, Lundeberg T, Cajander S, *et al.* 2003.

[34] Gnessi L, Fabbri A, Spera G. 1997.

[35] Seidl K, Holstein A-F. Evidence for the presence of nerve growth factor (NGF) and NGF receptors in human testis. Cell Tissue Res 1990; 261(3): 549-54.
[http://dx.doi.org/10.1007/BF00313534] [PMID: 2173974]

[36] Klein R. Role of neurotrophins in mouse neuronal development. FASEB J 1994; 8(10): 738-44.
[http://dx.doi.org/10.1096/fasebj.8.10.8050673] [PMID: 8050673]

CHAPTER 9

Integrated Treatment in Male Infertility

Abstract: While Western medicine is based on the paradigm of "one gene, one disease, one drug" and has a reductionistic approach, Chinese medicine is based on functional relationships, and evaluates the patient's pattern of signs and symptoms. Integration of Chinese medicine into Western medicine may be based on changes in sperm number, motility or morphology correlated to diagnostic patterns of TCM syndrome differentiation.

The obstructive azoospermias may be secondary to Blood, Phlegm or Dampness stagnation or Heat that blocks the sperm channel. The non-obstructive azoospermias are secondary to Kidney and Liver problems. The decrease in sperm motility may depend on problems in the Sperm Chamber, which is not heated when there is Qi deficiency, or is disturbed by Dampness and Heat. At the base of oligozoospermia there may be a deficiency of congenital Kidney Jing, or sexual excesses which consume Jing, or a Spleen deficiency which then fails to recharge the Kidney, or Perverse energies affecting the Sperm Chamber and causing infertility.

Keywords: Blood Stasis, Damp-Heat, Diagnosis, Integrated, Integration, Jing, Kidney Yin, Kidney Yang, Macroscopic, Microscopic, Paradigm, Pattern, Phlegm, Qi, Reductionistic, Spleen Qi, Stagnation, Stasis, Syndrome Differentiation, Systems Medicine.

It is difficult to integrate knowledge systems and medical approaches with different, almost opposite, conceptual and theoretical backgrounds. Western medicine is based on the paradigm of "one gene, one disease, one drug". Its reductionistic approach, which identifies the building blocks of life through the analysis of progressively smaller events and structures (Yin characteristics), has been the most commonly used approach for investigating biological phenomena. It is based on the belief that the ultimate causes of the observed behaviour of a system must be examined at the most fundamental level, and that the observable facts are consequences of laws deposited in the microscopic world. This paradigm has been used successfully in many investigations, but it has also been recognized that the knowledge of the molecular building blocks of a phenomenon does not necessarily guarantee a comprehension of that phenomenon. It is very clear for example that the medical diagnosis, done at the macroscopic properties of an incredibly complex system, is much more reliable than the results of the analysis of the single genes, receptors, or metabolites involved in the corresponding disease.

On the other hand Chinese medicine is based on functional relationships (Yang characteristics), and evaluates the patient's pattern of signs and symptoms, because the treatment is selected according to the type of imbalance in the patient. Its emergence approach, as opposed to the reductionistic approach, defines the principles as arising from the correlation properties of the groups of elements. This means that the properties of the system are not already present at the microscopic level, and the optimal vantage point for discovering those properties is not at the microscopic level but at the level of the system as a whole [1].

Integration of Chinese medicine into Western medicine is happening in part because of the accumulating evidence for its effectiveness, which has led to an increased demand by patients. On other levels, in Western medicine the crisis of the current paradigm is leading to a more widespread acceptance of the network metaphor, leading to a more holistic approach, at least in the basic sciences. Due to globalization and the migration of Chinese medicine to other social and cultural contexts, Chinese medicine has also been enriched by the tools and techniques of Western medicine. Today, TCM is not that of the Tang or Song or Ming era, for during the last century, while other traditional medicines have declined or disappeared altogether, it has combined elements from Western medicine. Already in 1932 the famous physician Shu Jin Mo had incorporated anatomy, physiology, bacteriology and general pathology in the curriculum of his school of TCM.

Modern TCM can be used to treat male infertility, and may even include a diagnosis based on the seminal fluid examination. Any changes in sperm number, motility or morphology may refer to diagnostic patterns of TCM syndrome differentiation. The correct syndrome differentiation allows the administration of an effective therapy in an exquisitely individualized approach, based on medical history, pulse, and tongue physical examination data. In this way an Integrated Medicine for male infertility is configured, which maximizes the contributions of both Chinese and Western Medicine. It is an Integrated Medicine, which serves to prevent the fragmentation of the medical culture which creates ineffective ghettos, and to enrich health care with a person-oriented model. In the field of male infertility this integration is literally at the seminal stages, as there are no published scientific studies in the English language evaluating the effectiveness and the efficacy of the combination of Chinese and Western Medicine in infertile men.

We describe below the integrated treatment of the main pathologic changes in the spermiogram.

AZOOSPERMIA

Pathogenesis

The obstructive azoospermias are secondary to Blood, Phlegm or Dampness stagnation or Heat that blocks the sperm channel. In these cases, it is necessary to consider first surgical treatment, and then a medical treatment with Western medicine and TCM. TCM can activate Blood and remove Blood stasis and is often very effective.

The non-obstructive azoospermias are secondary to Kidney and Liver problems. A congenital Jing deficiency or lack of nourishment of Jing can cause a deficiency of Kidney Yin and Kidney Yang, which results in lack of production of sperm. Also the Kidney Qi deficiency can alter the development of various parts of the male genital system. The effects can vary from the inability to produce semen, to oligozoospermia to normozoospermia, but with the inability to eject sperm from an obstruction at the level of the seminal tract.

The failure of Jing nourishment can be due to malnutrition, environmental problems (*e.g.* working at high temperatures), or testicular infections such as mumps (where Heat and toxins damage the collaterals, injuring sperm production).

Differential Diagnosis

Kidney Yang Deficiency

The signs and symptoms include light and cold semen, decreased volume of ejaculate up to anejaculation; decreased sex drive; chilliness, cold limbs, easily tired, weakness; low back pain and knee pain; clear and abundant urine, loose stools; the Tongue is pale, with white coating, the Pulse is weak (Ruo) and deep (Chen).

Treatment

Modified *Bu Tian Yu Ling Dan* (Tonify Heaven, Raise Boy Pill)

Rou Gui	10g	(Cortex Cinnamomi Cassiae)
Tu Si Zi	10g	(Semen Cuscutae Chinensis)
Rou Cong Rong	10g	(Herba Cistanches Deserticolae)

Shu Di Huang	20g	(Radix Rehmanniae Glutinosae Preparata)
Gou Qi Zi	10g	(Fructus Lycii)
Mu Dan Pi	10g	(Cortex Moutan Radicis)
Dang Shen	15g	(Radix Codonopsis Pilosulae)
Bai Zhu	10g	(Rhizoma Atractylodis Macrocephalae)
Ze Xie	10g	(Rhizoma Alismatis Orientalis)
Che Qian Zi	10g	(Semen Plantaginis)
Sheng Yu Rou	10g	(Fructus Corni Officinalis)
Wu Wei Zi	6g	(Fructus Schisandrae Chinensis)
Fu Ling	10g	(Sclerotium Poriae Cocos)

The decoction can be administered for 10 days. If after 10 days there has been no improvement, further cycles can be prescribed for a maximum period of six months. The subject should be monitored for side effects every 10 days in the first month, then once a month.

Kidney Yin Deficiency with Empty Heat

Seminal volume is much decreased, while density is increased. Ejaculation is weak (dripping). The causes can be congenital or acquired (sexual excesses or excessive mental stress). The signs and symptoms include increased sexual desire, low back pain, knee pain, memory problems, thirst, insomnia, hyperonirism. The Tongue has a thin or absent and Fine (Xi) Pulse, while the release of Empty Heat is manifested by red Tongue and Rapid (Shuo) Pulse.

Treatment

Modified **Shen Sui Yu Lin Dan** (Elixir to promote the production of sperm)

Rou Cong Rong	10g	(Herba Cistanches Deserticolae)
Tu Si Zi	10g	(Semen Cuscutae Chinensis)
Shu Di Huang	20g	(Radix Rehmanniae Glutinosae Preparata)
Gou Qi Zi	10g	(Fructus Lycii)
Sheng Yu Rou	10g	(Fructus Corni Officinalis)
He Shou Wu	10g	(Radix Polygoni Multiflori)
Dang Shen	15g	(Radix Codonopsis Pilosulae)
Bai Zhu	10g	(Rhizoma Atractylodis Macrocephalae)
Shan Yao	15g	(Radix Dioscoreae Oppositae)
Shen Qu	10g	(Massa Medica Fermentata)
Mai Ya	10g	(Fructus Hordei Vulgaris Germinatus)

With acupuncture it is possible to needle **CV4** (Guanyuan), **BL23** (Shenshu), **BL52** (Zhishi), **KI3** (Taixi), **BL20** (Pishu), **SP6** (Sanyinjiao). In the presence of Yang deficiency it is also possible to needle **GV4** (Mingmen) and **KI7** (Fuliu) with needle and moxa, and if there is excessive mental stress **BL15** (Xinshu) and **HT7** (Shenmen) can be treated.

Blood Stasis Blocks the Channel

There may be a history of trauma or surgery in the pelvic area. The volume of ejaculate is decreased. Other signs and symptoms include pain in the lower abdomen and genitals. There may be no other symptoms. The Tongue is purple and dark with bruises, the Pulse is Deep (Chen) and Choppy (Se). In this context, TCM is particularly effective.

Treatment

Modified *Xie Fu Zhu Yu Tang* (Decoction to Eliminate Stasis in the House of Blood)

Tao Ren	10g	(Semen Pruni Persicae)
Hong Hua	10g	(Flos Carthami Tinctorii)
Dan Shen	10g	(Radix Salviae Miltiorrhizae)
E Zhu	10g	(Rhizoma Curcumae Ezhu)
Niu Xi	10g	(Radix Cyathulae Officinalis)
Dang Gui Wei	10g	(Radix Angelicae Sinensis, estremità)
Chai Hu	6g	(Radix Bupleuri)
Zhi Ke	6g	(Fructus Citri Aurantii)
Chuan Xiong	10g	(Radix Ligustici Wallichii)
Shu Di Huang	15g	(Radix Rehmanniae Glutinosae)
Fu Ling	10g	(Sclerotium Poriae Cocos)
Bai Zhu	10g	(Rhizoma Atractylodis Macrocephalae)
Shen Qu	6g	(Massa Medica Fermentata)
Gan Cao	6g	(Radix Glycyrrhizae Uralensis)

Damp-Heat, Phlegm and Stasis Block the Channel

Generally the picture is associated with inflammation and infection of the urinary and/or genital tract. Semen volume is decreased and piospermia can be present. Other signs and symptoms include palpable masses in the pelvic area, dark and turbid urine, dysuria and difficulty urinating. The Tongue is red with a yellow greasy coating, the Pulse is Rapid (Shuo) and Slippery (Hua). In this context, TCM is particularly effective.

Treatment

Modified *Wu Shen Tang* (Five-Miracle Decoction) and modified *Xiao Luo Wan* (Scrophularia and Fritillaria Pill)

Che Qian Zi	10g	(Semen Plantaginis)
Sheng Yi Ren	15g	(Semen Coicis Lachryma-Jobi)
Yin Hua	10g	(Flos Lonicerae Japonicae)
Tu Fu Ling	10g	(Rhizoma Smilacis Glabrae)
Gan Cao	6g	(Radix Glycyrrhizae Uralensis)
Chuan Niu Xi	15g	(Radix Cyathulae Officinalis)
Yi Mu Cao	10g	(Herba Leonuri Heterophylli)
Bei Mu	12g	(Bulbus Fritillariae)
Xuan Shen	15g	(Radix Scrophulariae Ningpoensis)
Shi Chang Pu	6g	(Rhizoma Acori)

ASTHENOZOOSPERMIA

Pathogenesis

The decrease in sperm motility may depend on problems in the Sperm Chamber, which is not heated when there is Qi deficiency, or is disturbed by Dampness and Heat. The Qi which warms the Sperm Chamber is activated by the Kidney Jing. Both the Kidney Qi and the Kidney Jing can be deficient from congenital causes or due to excessive consumption. The Middle Burner is a source of Qi and Blood, which produce sperm; at this level other causes of asthenozoospermia can be found. Dampness and Heat directly damage sperm.

In cases of trauma, inflammation of the prostate or varicose spermatic veins there can be a blockage of the Collaterals with a non-harmonic circulation of Blood and Qi, which do not arrive to nourish sperm.

In case of asthenozoospermia it is possible to needle **KI6** (Zhao Hai) and **GV4** (Ming Men) to tonify Kidney Yang.

Differential Diagnosis

Kidney Qi Deficiency

The signs and symptoms include hypoactive sexual desire and impotence or premature ejaculation; there will be fatigue, polyuria with clear urine, low back pain and knee pain, loose stools. Alterations in semen analysis will be correlated to Yang deficiency: asthenozoospermia, presence of immature elements (in Yin deficiency there is teratozoospermia). The Tongue is pale with white coating, the Pulse is Deep (Ruo), Fine (Xi) and Weak (Chen).

Treatment

Modified Huang *Jing Zan Yu Dan* (Special Pill to Aid Fertility) and modified *Wu Zi Yan Zong Wan* (Five Seed Progeny Pill, or Five Ancestors Pill)

Huang Jing	10g	(Rhizoma Polygonati)
Tu Si Zi	10g	(Semen Cuscutae Chinensis)
Yin Yang Huo	10g	(Herba Epimedii)
Chuan Duan	10g	(Radix Dipsaci Asperi)
Gou Qi Zi	10g	(Fructus Lycii)
Wu Wei Zi	6g	(Fructus Schisandrae Chinensis)
Shu Di Huang	15g	(Radix Rehmanniae Glutinosae Praeparata)
Dang Shen	15g	(Radix Codonopsis Pilosulae)
Bai Zhu	10g	(Rhizoma Atractylodis Macrocephalae)
Dang Gui	10g	(Radix Angelicae Sinensis)
Che Qian Zi	10g	(Semen Plantaginis)
Gan Cao	6g	(Radix Glycyrrhizae Uralensis)

Kidney Jing Deficiency

The signs and symptoms include feeling of light-headedness, insomnia, forgetfulness, mild tinnitus; if there is a serious deficiency, there will be more Fire, so there will be increased sexual desire, premature ejaculation, dark yellow urine. The Tongue may be red (if there is release of Heat) and with thin coating, the Pulse is Fine (Xi) and Rapid (Shuo).

Treatment

Modified *Qi Bao Mei Ran Dan* (Seven-Treasure Special Pill for Beautiful Whiskers)

Shu Di Huang	15g	(Radix Rehmanniae Glutinosae Praeparata)
Zhi Shou Wu	10g	(Radix Polygoni Multiflori Praeparata)
Gou Qi Zi	10g	(Fructus Lycii)
Tu Si Zi	10g	(Semen Cuscutae Chinensis)
Bu Gu Zhi	10g	(Fructus Psoraleae Corylifoliae)
Niu Xi	10g	(Radix Achyranthis Bidentatae)

Chuan Duan	10g	(Radix Dipsaci Asperi)
Fu Ling	10g	(Sclerotium Poriae Cocos)
Che Qian Zi	6g	(Semen Plantaginis)
Hong Zao	10g	(Fructus Jujubae)
Mu Xiang	6g	(Radix Aucklandiae)
Mai Ya	6g	(Fructus Hordei Germinatus)
Shen Qu	6g	(Massa Medica Fermentata)

Spleen and Stomach Deficiency. The signs and symptoms include asthenozoospermia, poor appetite, abdominal distension, loose stools, fatigue, weak constitution, sallow complexion. The Tongue is enlarged with dental markings and with thin coating, the Pulse is Fine (Xi).

Treatment

Modified **Bu Zhong Yi Qi Tang** (Tonify the Middle and Augment the Qi Decoction)

Dang Shen	15g	(Radix Codonopsis)
Huang Qi	15g	(Radix Astragali Membranacei)
Bai Zhu	10g	(Rhizoma Atractylodis Macrocephalae)
Dang Gui	10g	(Radix Angelicae Sinensis)
Gou Qi Zi	10g	(Fructus Lycii)
Fu Ling	10g	(Sclerotium Poriae Cocos)
Ge Gen	6→10g	(Radix Puerariae)
Chao Mai Ya	6g	(Fructus Hordei Vulgaris Germinatus)
Chao Gu Ya	6g	(Fructus Oryzae Sativae Germinatus)
Gan Cao	6g	(Radix Glycyrrhizae)

Damp-Heat blocks the Lower Burner. The signs and symptoms include turbid semen, piospermia, turbid urine, dysuria with burning pain, bitter mouth, wet genitals with a feeling of prolapse of the genital organs. The Tongue is red with a yellow, thickened and sticky coating, the Pulse is Rapid (Shuo) and Slippery (Hua) or Wiry (Xian).

Treatment

Modified **Bei Xie Fen Qing Yin** (Dioscorea Hypoglauca Decoction to Separate the Clear)

Bei Xie	15g	(Rhizoma Dioscoreae Hypoglaucae)
Wu Yao	10g	(Radix Linderae Strychnifoliae)
Shi Chang Pu	6g	(Rhizoma Acori)
Tu Si Zi	10g	(Semen Cuscutae Chinensis)
Yi Yi Ren	15g	(Semen Coicis Lachryma-Jobi)
Fu Ling	10g	(Sclerotium Poriae Cocos)
Shan Yao	15g	(Radix Dioscoreae Oppositae)
Tu Fu Ling	10→15g	(Rhizoma Smilacis Glabrae)
Yu Xing Cao	10→15g	(Herba Houttuyniae)

Formula ***Bi Yu San****: Hua Shi* (Talcum), *Gan Cao* (Radix Glycyrrhizae Uralensis), *Qing Dai* (Indigo Pulverata Levis)

Obstruction of the Collaterals

The signs and symptoms include asthenozoospermia, oligozoospermia, hematospermia (secondary to Blood stasis overflowing out of the Channels), feeling of pelvic distention and prolapse; the prostate has increased consistency and nodules on palpation. The Tongue is dark red with bruises on both sides, the Pulse is Fine (Xi) and Choppy (Se).

Treatment

Modified ***Tao Hong Si Wu Tang*** (Four-Substance Decoction with Safflower and Peach Pit)

Tao Ren	10g	(Semen Pruni Persicae)
Hong Hua	10g	(Flos Carthami Tinctorii)
Shu Di Huang	10g	(Radix Rehmanniae Glutinosae Praeparata)
Dang Gui	10g	(Radix Angelicae Sinensis)
Chuan Xiong	10g	(Radix Ligustici Wallichii)
Dan Shen	10g	(Radix Salviae Miltiorrhizae)
Yi Mu Cao	10g	(Herba Leonuri Heterophylli)
Gan Cao	6g	(Radix Glycyrrhizae Uralensis)

AUTOIMMUNE INFERTILITY

Pathogenesis

The presence of any type of autoantibody is related to the constitution of the individual, as it may be secondary to a deficiency of congenital Jing Qi, which leads to a deficiency of Yin and Spleen Qi.

Antisperm antibodies (ASA) can be found in sperm or in the blood serum. The presence of ASA in the sperm derives from a local reaction and it can damage the sperm; if they are present in the serum this is due to a dysfunction of the immune system.

Several causes can help create an autoimmune dysfunction, and Western medicine has identified several of them (alcohol abuse, excessive sexual activity, smoking, *etc.*). In TCM, ASA are mainly due to Perverse Energy (especially Dampness, Heat and Blood stasis) prevailing on the correct energy (Zheng Qi). These Perverse Energies are often complex factors in different relationships with each other, so that one (or more than one) may be primarily responsible for the disease. Zheng Qi is supported by the Spleen, the Lung and the Kidney.

The goal of treatment is to negativize the ASA, particularly in the seminal fluid. This goal is easier to achieve and more effective for the re-establishment of fertility than the elimination of ASA in the serum.

The treatment of autoimmune infertility with acupuncture consists of tonifying the Liver and the Kidney, invigorating the Blood and freeing the Collaterals with a basic protocol that must be done daily for two months. The points used are: **BL18** (Ganshu), **LR3** (Taichong), **BL23** (Shenshu), **KI3** (Taixi), **BL15** (Xinshu), **HT7** (Shenmen), **BL17** (Geshu), **SP10** (Xuehai), **BL22** (Sanjiaoshu), **TE4** (Yangchi).

The basic treatment of autoimmune infertility with TCM is to tonify Zheng Qi and expel the Perverse Energy. There are two possibilities; either it is the local disease that affects the whole body, or it is the body that influences the local part. The therapy will be different in the two cases. In the first case we must expel the Perverse Energies, and then supplement and tonify Zheng Qi, while in the second case we must supplement and tonify Zheng Qi, and then expel the Perverse Energies. These two options can be differentiated by a thorough history, while it is difficult to differentiate them through the Tongue and Pulse, because sometimes they give wrong information. For example in the case of an alcoholic with a pattern of Damp-Heat and a red Tongue with yellow greasy coating, but with fatigue, this will be a pattern of deficiency.

These are the herbs commonly used in the two protocols:

Qu Xie (expel the Perverse Energies)

Ye Ju Hua	15g	(Flos Chrysanthemi Indici)
Bai Jiang Cao	10g	(Herba cum Radix Patriniae)

Cheng Teng	20g	(Caulis et Folium Hederae)
Jin Yin Hua	10g	(Flos Lonicerae Japonicae)
Tu Fu Ling	15g	(Rhizoma Smilacis Glabrae)
Chuan Niu Xi	10g	(Radix Cyathulae Officinalis)

Fu Zheng (tonify Zheng Qi)

Huang Qi	15→20g	(Radix Astragali Membranacei)
Dang Gui	10g	(Radix Angelicae Sinensis)
Tai Zi Shen	15g	(Radix Pseudostellariae)
Huang Jing	10g	(Rhizoma Polygonati)
Chao Bai Shao	10g	(Radix Paeoniae Lactiflorae)
Tian Hua Fen	10→15g	(Radix Trichosanthis Kirilowii)
Wu Wei Zi	6→10g	(Fructus Schisandrae)

Note that often the dispersing recipes are also in part tonifying, whereas here in the first protocol (Qu Xie, expel Perverse Energies) the herbs are only dispersing.

Differential Diagnosis

Yin Deficiency with Yin Fire

The signs and symptoms include strong sexual desire, premature ejaculation or anejaculation during sexual activity, sometimes hemospermia; positivity (+ or ++) in serum of antibodies against sperm, other autoantibodies can also be present; irritability, thirst, insomnia, hyperonirism, low back pain and knee pain, constipation, dark urine, dysuria. The Tongue is red with a thin coating, the Pulse is Fine (Xi) and Fast (Shuo).

Treatment

Modified **Dang Gui Liu Huang Tang** (Angelica and Six-Yellow Decoction)

Dang Gui	10g	(Radix Angelicae Sinensis)
Sheng Di Huang	15g	(Radix Rehmanniae Glutinosae)
Shu Di Huang	15g	(Radix Rehmanniae Glutinosae Praeparata)
Huang Qin	10g	(Radix Scutellariae Baicalensis)
Huang Bai	10g	(Cortex Phellodendri)
Chao Bai Shao	10g	(Radix Paeoniae Lactiflorae)
Chao Mu Dan Pi	10g	(Cortex Moutan Radicis)
Shou Wu	10g	(Radix Polygoni Multiflori)

| *Gan Cao* | 6g | (Radix Glycyrrhizae Uralensis) |
| *Tu Fu Ling* | 10g | (Rhizoma Smilacis Glabrae) |

Obstruction of the Collaterals and the Sperm Cannot Get Out

The history reveals an obvious trauma and/or surgery in the pelvic area. The signs and symptoms include masses in the epididymis and/or in the testes, distention and pain in the lower abdomen, in the prostate and in the epididymis. The Tongue is dark red with bruising, the Pulse is Fine (Xi) and Choppy (Se).

Treatment

Modified ***Tuo Li Xiao Du San*** (Support the Interior and Eliminate Toxin Powder)

Sheng Huang Qi	15g	(Radix Astragali Membranacei)
Dang Gui	10g	(Radix Angelicae Sinensis)
Bai Zhu	10g	(Rhizoma Atractylodis Macrocephalae)
Bai Shao	10g	(Radix Paeoniae Lactiflorae)
Chuan Xiong	10g	(Radix Ligustici Wallichii)
Tian Hua Fen	10g	(Radix Trichosanthis Kirilowii)
Hong Hua	10g	(Flos Carthami Tinctorii)
Tao Ren	10g	(Semen Pruni Persicae)
Gan Cao	6g	(Radix Glycyrrhizae Uralensis)
Shen Qu	10g	(Massa Medica Fermentata)
Hong Zao	10g	(Fructus Jujubae)

Spleen and Qi Wei Deficiency

The Spleen plays a central role in the production of Blood, and controls the use of the nutrients that are vital for a healthy immune response, involving the neuro-endocrine-immune system. Wei Qi has a defence, surveillance and tolerance function, and corresponds to the immune system. In particular the tolerance function of the immune system can recognize self from non-self and prevents autoimmune diseases. Wei Qi is damaged by Dampness, which can be produced in case of Spleen deficiency. The signs and symptoms of this syndrome include easy susceptibility to disease, appetite loss, fatigue, easily tired, paleness, soft stools. The Tongue is pale with white coating and dental markings, the Pulse is Fine (Xi) and Weak (Xu).

Treatment

Modified ***Yu Ping San*** (Jade Windscreen Powder) and modified ***Shen Ling Bai Zhu San*** (Ginseng, Poria and Atractylodes Powder)

Sheng Huang Qi	15g	(Radix Astragali Membranacei)
Bai Zhu	10g	(Rhizoma Atractylodis Macrocephalae)
Fang Feng	6g	(Radix Saposhnikoviae)
Tai Zi Shen	15g	(Radix Pseudostellariae)
Huang Jing	10g	(Rhizoma Polygonati)
Shan Yao	15g	(Radix Dioscoreae)
Fu Ling	10g	(Sclerotium Poriae Cocos)
Chao Bai Shao	10g	(Radix Paeoniae Lactiflorae)
Gan Cao	6g	(Radix Glycyrrhizae)
Da Zao	10g	(Fructus Jujubae)

Damp-Heat. The signs and symptoms include yellow and sticky sperm, with piospermia; bitter taste in the mouth, thirst without desire to drink, dark urine, Lower Urinary Tract Symptoms (LUTS), dysuria, sense of contraction and pain when urinating. The Tongue is red with a yellow greasy coating, the Pulse is Slippery (Hua) and Fast (Shuo) or Wiry (Xian).

Treatment

Modified *Wu Shen Tang* (Five-Miracle Decoction)

Sheng Yi Yi Ren	15g	(Semen Coicis Lachryma-Jobi)
Che Qian Zi	10g	(Semen Plantaginis)
Fu Ling	10g	(Sclerotium Poriae Cocos)
Jin Yin Hua	10g	(Flos Lonicerae Japonicae)
Ye Ju Hua	15g	(Flos Chrysanthemi Indici)
Zi Hua Di Ding	10g	(Herba cum Rd Violae Yedoensitis)
Yi Mu Cao	10g	(Herba Leonuri Heterophylli)
Chuan Niu Xi	10g	(Radix Cyathulae Officinalis)
Sheng Gan Cao	6g	(Radix Glycyrrhizae Uralensis)
Shen Qu	10g	(Massa Medica Fermentata)
Hong Zao	10g	(Fructus Jujubae)

OLIGOZOOSPERMIA

Pathogenesis

This is an abnormality of the seminal fluid that is dependent on the Kidney, the Spleen and the Liver, and that affects the Sperm Chamber. At the base of oligozoospermia there may be a deficiency of congenital Kidney Jing, or sexual excesses which consume Jing, or a Spleen deficiency which then fails to recharge the Kidney, or Perverse energies affecting the Sperm Chamber and causing infertility.

Differential Diagnosis

Kidney Jing Deficiency

Kidney Jing may be impaired because of a congenital deficiency, or it can be consumed directly from sexual excesses or from the Heat generated from foods that are too Hot, too Dry or too Spicy.

The signs and symptoms include low-volume, clear and watery ejaculation; premature aging, greying hair; presence of vertigo, tinnitus, insomnia, difficulty in maintaining concentration, poor memory, lumbar and knee soreness that occurs or worsens with minimal efforts. The Tongue is small, red and with thin coating, the Pulse is Fine (Xi) and Fast (Shuo).

Treatment

Modified *Ju Jing Tang* (Decoction to support Jing)

Shu Di Huang	12g	(Radix Rehmanniae Glutinosae Praeparata)
Zhi Shou Wu	12g	(Radix Polygoni Multiflori Praeparata)
Gou Qi Zi	12g	(Fructus Lycii)
Tu Si Zi	10g	(Semen Cuscutae Chinensis)
Yin Yang Huo	10g	(Herba Epimedii)
Tai Zi Shen	12g	(Radix Pseudostellariae)
Fu Ling	12g	(Sclerotium Poriae Cocos)
Huang Jing	12g	(Rhizoma Polygonati)
Fu Pen Zi	10g	(Fructus Rubi Chingii)
Che Qian Zi	10g	(Semen Plantaginis)

Kidney Yang Deficiency

The subject with Kidney Yang deficiency fails to warm the Kidneys and the Sperm Chamber, so sperm cannot mature. The syndrome may be due to overwork, to chronic diseases, to sexual excess, or too much intake of Cold foods.

The signs and symptoms include shortness of breath, fatigue, cold extremities, low back pain and knee pain, frequent urination, nocturnal enuresis, clear polyuria, loose stools. The Tongue is pale with white coating, the Pulse is Weak (Ruo) and Deep (Chen).

Treatment

Modified *Wu Zi Yan Zong* (Five Seed Progeny Pill, or Five Ancestors Pill) and modified *You Gui Wan* (Restore the Right Kidney Pill)

Fu Zi	6g	(Radix Aconiti Carmichaeli Praeparata)
Rou Gui	10g	(Cortex Cinnamomi Cassiae)
Shu Di Huang	15g	(Radix Rehmanniae Glutinosae Praeparata)
Dang Gui	10g	(Radix Angelicae Sinensis)
Sheng Yu Rou	10g	(Fructus Corni Officinalis)
Tu Si Zi	10g	(Semen Cuscutae Chinensis)
Gou Qi Zi	10g	(Fructus Lycii)
Du Zhong	10g	(Cortex Eucommiae Ulmoidis)
Gan Cao	6g	(Radix Glycyrrhizae Uralensis)

Spleen Qi Deficiency

This syndrome is usually due to poor lifestyle habits, including an improper diet, too much exposure to damp weather, or to chronic diseases, stress or worries. Spleen Qi deficiency leads to insufficient production of Blood; Blood and Jing are connected, so if the Blood is insufficient Jing also becomes insufficient.

The signs and symptoms include watery semen; fatigue, weakness, low sex drive, easy fatigue; poor digestion, loss of appetite, bloating after meals, soft stools. The Tongue is swollen, with white and moist coating, the Pulse is Fine (Xi).

Treatment

Modified *Bu Zhong Yi Qi Tang* (Tonify the Middle and Augment the Qi Decoction)

Ren Shen	10g	(Radix Ginseng)
Huang Qi	5g	(Radix Astragali Membranacei)
Bai Zhu	10g	(Rhizoma Atractylodis Macrocephalae)
Dang Gui	6g	(Radix Angelicae Sinensis)
Gou Qi Zi	10g	(Fructus Lycii)
Fu Ling	10g	(Sclerotium Poriae Cocos)
Chen Pi	6g	(Pericarpium Citri Reticulatae)

Tu Si Zi	10g	(Semen Cuscutae Chinensis)
Sha Yuan Zi	10g	(Semen Astragali Complanati)
Zhi Gan Cao	6g	(Radix Glycyrrhizae Uralensis)

Damp-Heat in the Lower Burner. Dampness and Heat generate from spicy, fat, heavy food, or penetrate from the Exterior if the weather is humid and/or hot. Dampness and Heat go downward along the meridians and interfere with the Sperm Chamber, causing a decrease in sperm count.

The signs and symptoms include decreased volume of ejaculate, painful ejaculation, murky yellow sperm, sometimes with piospermia, abnormal liquefaction, thirst without desire to drink, oliguria and with murky dark urine, dysuria, dry stool, wet genitals, genital itching, red eyes, irritability, bitter mouth. The Tongue has a yellow, thick and sticky coating, the Pulse is Rapid (Shuo) and Slippery (Hua).

Treatment

Modified ***Bei Xie Fen Qing Yin*** (Dioscorea Hypoglauca Decoction to Separate the Clear)

Bei Xie	105g	(Rhizoma Dioscoreae Hypoglaucae)
Wu Yao	8g	(Radix Linderae Strychnifoliae)
Shi Chang Pu	10g	(Rhizoma Acori)
Tu Si Zi	12g	(Semen Cuscutae Chinensis)
Yi Yi Ren	15g	(Semen Coicis Lachryma-Jobi)
Fu Ling	12g	(Sclerotium Poriae Cocos)
Che Qian Zi	10g	(Semen Plantaginis)

Qi Stagnation and Blood Stasis

The causes of Qi stagnation are usually emotional (anger, frustration, sadness, *etc.*), and if Qi stagnation is severe and/or prolonged, it leads to Blood stasis. Blood stasis can be caused also by Qi deficiency, trauma, surgery, bleeding, and Heat or Cold in the Blood.

The signs and symptoms include decreased ejaculate volume, hemospermia, increased time of liquefaction; perineal soreness and pain; irritability, depression, stress, sighs; bloating. The Tongue is purple, with petechiae, or bruising at the sides. The Pulse is Deep (Chen) and Choppy (Se).

Treatment

Modified *Xue Fu Zhu Yu Tang* (Drive Out Stasis in the Mansion of Blood Decoction)

Tao Ren	15g	(Semen Pruni Persicae)
Hong Hua	10g	(Flos Carthami Tinctorii)
Dan Shen	12g	(Radix Salviae Miltiorrhizae)
Chi Shao Yao	10g	(Radix Paeoniae Rubrae)
Dang Gui Wei	10g	(Radix Angelicae Sinensis)
Chai Hu	6g	(Radix Bupleuri)
Chuan Xiong	6g	(Radix Ligustici Wallichii)
Shu Di Huang	10g	(Radix Rehmanniae Glutinosae Praeparata)

ABNORMALITIES IN SEMEN LIQUEFACTION

The normal process of liquefaction of the ejaculate depends on the interaction between Kidney Jing and the heating activity of the Ministerial Fire *via* the transformation function of Qi (气化 Qi Hua). As mentioned in Chapter 5, the Ministerial Fire, *i.e.* the Kidney Yang, heats the water of the Kidney Yin (the Jing) and the liquids of the Lower Triple Burner. Alterations of liquefaction occur in the Sperm Chamber and may be related to Kidney Qi and Yin deficiency, or to the presence of Damp-Heat in the Lower Burner, or Empty Fire burning Jing.

Differential Diagnosis

Kidney Yin Deficiency

Kidney Yin deficiency can be either congenital, or secondary to stress or sexual excesses. The Yin deficiency causes a thickening of the sperm, which liquefies with difficulty. The Empty Fire can burn sperm.

The signs and symptoms include lengthening of the time of liquefaction, signs of Heat such as painful ejaculation, thickened semen, hemospermia, nocturnal emissions, premature ejaculation, dry mouth, warmth in the five centres, tinnitus, fatigue, insomnia. The Tongue is red with a thin yellow coating, the Pulse is Fine (Xi) and Rapid (Shuo).

Treatment

Modified *Zhi Bai Di Huang Wan* (Anemarrhena, Phellodendron and Rehmannia Pill)

Zhi Mu	10g	(Rhizoma Anemarrhenae Asphodeloidis)
Huang Bai	10g	(Cortex Phellodendri)
Shu Di Huang	15g	(Radix Rehmanniae Glutinosae Praeparata)
Shan Yao	10g	(Radix Dioscoreae Oppositae)
Fu Ling	10g	(Sclerotium Poriae Cocos)
Ze Xie	10g	(Rhizoma Alismatis Orientalis)
Mu Dan Pi	10g	(Cortex Moutan Radicis)
Tian Hua Fen	10g	(Radix Trichosanthis Kirilowii)
Chao Bai Shao	12g	(Radix Paeoniae Lactiflorae Praeparata)

Kidney Yang Deficiency

Kidney Yang deficiency can be congenital, or secondary to chronic diseases or to cosmopathogenic Cold or Damp invasion. Kidney deficiency leads to insufficient heating of the Ming Men and to abnormalities of liquefaction.

The signs and symptoms include very white semen, decreased sex drive, impotence, premature ejaculation, pale urination, nocturia, cold lumbar area. The Tongue has a thin white coating, the Pulse is Weak (Ruo) and Deep (Chen).

Treatment

Modified ***Ba Ji Er Xian Tang*** (Two Immortals Decoction)

Ba Ji Tian	10g	(Radix Morindae Officinalis)
Xian Mao	15g	(Rhizoma Curculiginis Orchioidis)
Yin Yang Huo	10g	(Herba Epimedii)
Gui Zhi	6g	(Ramulus Cinnamomi Cassiae)
Wang Bu Liu Xing	10g	(Semen Vaccariae Segetalis)
Shu Di Huang	12g	(Radix Rehmanniae Glutinosae Praeparata)
Wu Yao	8g	(Radix Linderae Strychnifoliae)
Shi Chang Pu	10g	(Rhizoma Acori)

Damp-Heat

Dampness and Heat can develop from the ingestion of Spicy, Hot and Damp foods, and from the invasion of External Heat and Dampness, that descend along the meridians and reach the Sperm Chamber.

The signs and symptoms include yellow and sticky ejaculate, wet scrotum, tenderness in the lower abdomen, dysuria, bitter mouth. The Tongue is red with a yellow greasy coating, the Pulse is Rapid (Shuo) and Slippery (Hua) or Wiry (Xian).

Treatment

Modified *Bei Xie Fen Qing Yin* (Dioscorea Hypoglauca Decoction to Separate the Clear)

Bei Xie	15g	(Rhizoma Dioscoreae Hypoglaucae)
Wu Yao	8g	(Radix Linderae Strychnifoliae)
Shi Chang Pu	6g	(Rhizoma Acori)
Tu Si Zi	12g	(Semen Cuscutae Chinensis)
Kun Bu	12g	(Thallus Laminariae seu Eckloniae)
Fu Ling	6g	(Sclerotium Poriae Cocos)
Huang Bai	10g	(Cortex Phellodendri)
Hai Zao	12g	(Herba Sargassii)

CONSENT FOR PUBLICATION

Not applicable.

CONFLICT OF INTEREST

The author (editor) declares no conflict of interest, financial or otherwise.

ACKNOWLEDGEMENT

Declared none.

BIBLIOGRAPHY

[1]   Conti F, Valerio MC, Zbilut JP, Giuliani A. Will systems biology offer new holistic paradigms to life sciences? Syst Synth Biol 2007; 1(4): 161-5.

Case Reports

Here we report some case studies from the experience in the Acupuncture Clinic for Male Infertility in the Complex Unit of Endocrinology, which was open from 2008 to 2011 at the CTO Hospital in Rome, Italy. To access the Clinic, men had to fulfil the following inclusion criteria:

• Inability to fertilize the partner after at least one year of attempts.

At least two pathologic spermiograms carried out at intervals of 4–6 weeks, with oligozoospermia, asthenozoospermia and/or teratozoospermia according to the WHO criteria.

The normality parameters according to the WHO criteria were:

• Normal count: > 20 million sperm/ml.
• Normal motility: > 50% with vigorous and progressive movement.
• Normal morphology: > 14% with normal forms.
• Negativity of endocrinological laboratory tests (LH, FSH, prolactin, estradiol, testosterone, thyroid, adrenal or other hormones).

Patients were excluded if they had been treated with androgens in the last 12 months, if they had severe systemic diseases, or recent antibiotic treatment (suspended for less than a month). Table **15** shows the baseline characteristics of the included subjects.

The acupuncture treatment was done using stainless steel, sterile and disposable needles (size 0.25 x 25 mm, Hwato), inserted for a depth of 5–10 mm depending on the location. The needles were left in situ for 25 min without manipulation and then removed.

In subjects with asthenozoospermia, the following points were treated for 4 weeks: **KI16, BL29, BL43** (needle and moxa), **BL53, GB41**.

In subjects with oligoasthenozoospermia, the above protocol was alternated with a protocol for oligozoospermia, consisting of the following points: **LI16, KI11, ST36, BL26-29-32**. These subjects were treated for 8 weeks. In the case of varicocele, the following points were added: **GB22** and **PC9**.

The data showed a significant increase in fast progressive motility in the second hour. The improvement is observed especially in men with atypical forms <70% (see Table **16**). This is in line with several studies published in the literature, most of which suggested an effect of acupuncture on spermatic motility without any effect on teratozoospermia.

Table 15. Basic characteristics of subjects prior to acupuncture treatment.

	CT	LD	AL	AM	SS	MC
Age (years)	38	39	44	39	41	37
Varicocele	Yes	Yes	Yes	No	Yes	No

(Table 15) contd.....

	CT	LD	AL	AM	SS	MC
Waist circumference (cm)	98	101	93	103	104	92
Smoker	Yes	No	No	No	No	No
Previous use of acupuncture	Yes	No	No	No	No	No

Table 16. Data on the number, motility and atypical forms in the seminal fluid before and after acupuncture.

	Sperm Count (M/mL)		Fast Progressive Motility 2^ h (%)		Atypical Forms (%)	
	Before	After	Before	After	Before	After
CT	5	3	0	0	96	99
LD	11	13	18.8	25.9	76	72
AL	7	4	0	0	96	99
AM	78	32	18.8	27.9	67	67
SS	0.2	5	0	2.3	99	92
CM	43	32	20.9	25.8	64	62
Mean	*24*	*14.8*	*9.7*	*13.6*	*83*	*81.8*
P value		*0.28*		*0.05*		*0.44*

No side effects of acupuncture have been observed, except for rare minor bleeding episodes at the needle insertion site.

Appendix

APPENDIX 1

GENETIC TESTING IN MALE INFERTILITY

Clinical condition	Genetic test	Genetic diagnosis	Actions
Non-obstructive azoospermia	Karyotype	Klinefelter syndrome	Cryopreservation in young age, ev. TESE
Severe oligozoospermia (<10M/mL)		Robertsonian translocations	Counselling (offspring with Down or Patau syndrome)
Poliabortivity		Reciprocal translocations	Counselling (increase of fetal mortality)
Family history of hypogonadotropic hypogonadism		Inversions	Counselling (offspring with duplications or chromosomal deficits)
Non-obstructive azoospermia	Y Chromosome-microdeletions	AZFa microdeletion	Sertoli Cells Only syndrome, TESE is contraindicated
Severe oligozoospermia (<5M/mL in the non-idiopathic forms and <10 M/mL in the idiopathic forms)		AZFb microdeletion	Spermatogenic arrest, TESE is contraindicated
		AZFc microdeletion	Cryopreservation in young age, TESE, deletion transmitted to male offspring
Obstructive azoospermia	CFTR gene mutations	Cystic fibrosis	TESA and in vitro fertilization
Agenesis of the vas deferens			
Severe alterations of the spermiogram	gr/gr deletion	gr/gr deletion	Risk of testicular cancer, deletion transmitted to male offspring

APPENDIX 2

FORMULAS FOR TREATING MALE INFERTILITY WITH TRADITIONAL CHINESE MEDICINE

Kidney Yin Deficiency

- *Wuzi Yanzong Wan and Zuogui Wan*
- *Liu Wei Di Huang Wan*
- *Zhi Bai Di Huang Wan*

Kidney Yang Deficiency

- *You Gui Wan*
- *Jin Gui Shen Qi*
- *Gui Ling Ji*

Kidney Qi Deficiency

- *Shen Bao*
- *Shen Qi Da Bu Wan*

Kidney Jing Deficiency

- *Wuzi Yanzong Wan*
- *Nan Xing Bu Shen Fang*

Deficiency of Spleen Qi and Heart Blood

- *Ba Zhen Sheng Jing Tang*
- *Ren Shen Gui Pi Wan*

Liver Qi Stagnation

- *Xiao Yao San*

Liver Blood Stasis

- *Xue Fu Zhu Yu Tang*

Damp-Heat Accumulation in the Lower Burner

- *Bei Xie Shen Shi Tang*
- *Bei Xie Fen Qing Tang*
- *Long Dan Xie Gan Tang*

Phlegm and Blood Stasis Blocking the Passage of Essence

- *Cang Fu Dao Tan Tang*

APPENDIX 3

Acupoint	Action	Symptoms
CV13 **Shang Guan** 上脘 **Upper Stomach Cavity**	First separation of clear from turbid material at the level of the Stomach	Does not digest some foods, epigastric bloating after meals, frontal headache after meals, stagnation of liquids in the stomach, logorrhea, and inability to choose what is needed and to let go of what is not necessary
CV11 **Jian Li** 建里 **Establish Mile**	Second separation of clear from turbid material at the level of the Small Intestine	Abdominal bloating or frontal headache after meals, logorrhea
SI1 **Shao Ze** 少澤 **Lesser Marsh**	Separation of Pure from Impure at the level of the Small Intestine and transport to the Kidney	Urticaria from food
SP6 **San Yin Jiao** 三陰交 **Meeting of the 3 Yin**	Ascent to the Lung	Presence of Dampness in the Lower Burner
GB38 **Yang Fu** 陽輔 **Support of Yang**	Diaphragm blocked by Damp-Heat	Bitter mouth in the morning
BL17 Ge Shu 膈俞 **Diaphragm Shu** **BL46 Ge Guan** 膈關 **Diaphragm Pass,** **CV17 Shan Zhong** 膻中 **Chest Centre**	Blocked Diaphragm	Epigastric pain and/or hiccups
GV9 **Zhi Yang** 至陽 **Arrival of Yang**	Blocked Diaphragm	Anxiety and panic attacks
LR10 **Zu Wu Li** 足五里 **Foot Five Li**	Blocked Diaphragm	Dyspepsia; anger
LR5 **Li Gou** 蠡溝 **Worm Groove**	Blocked Diaphragm; Luo connecting point	Gynecological problems (ovarian cysts or uterine fibroids)
LI14 **Bi Nao** 臂臑 **Shoulder Joint**	The Lung moves down Blood and Lung Shen (Po); Reunion point of ST, LI and Yang Wei Mai channels	Infertility, bereavement and separations; sensitive to injustice, excessively tidy; bronchial asthma, bronchitis

(Contd.....)

Acupoint	Action	Symptoms
LI15 **Jian Yu 肩髃** **Shoulder Bone**	The Lung moves down Wei Qi; Origin of the LI distinct channel; Reunion point with Yang Qiao Mai	Decreased libido, depression, lower back pain due to herniated disks
LI16 **Ju Gu 巨骨** **Great Bone**	The Lung moves down the Ye Fluids to the Lower Burner Reunion point with Yang Qiao Mai; Upper Sea of the Marrows	Bronchial asthma, bronchitis, phlegm; tremors, epilepsy;
KI11 **Heng Gu 横骨** **Pubic Bone**	The Yin Kidney grasps the turbid Ye Fluids to nourish the Marrows (Gao); Reunion point with Chong Mai	Post-prandial fatigue; weight gain; stagnation of turbid Ye Fluids in the lower burner with LUTS and diarrhea
KI12 **Da He 大赫** **Great Manifestation**	Disposal of the turbid Ye Fluids by the Urinary Bladder; nourishment of the Bao; Reunion point with Chong Mai	Frequent cystitis, urinary frequency, dysuria
KI13 **Qi Xue 氣穴** **Qi Hole**	Disposal of the turbid Ye Fluids by the Small Intestine; nourishment of the Bao; Reunion point with Chong Mai	Post-prandial fatigue; LUTS
KI14 **Si Man 四滿** **Fourfold Fullness**	Disposal of the turbid Ye Fluids by the Lower Burner; Reunion point with Chong Mai	Alterations of the lower orifices (proctitis, cystitis, *etc*); fluid retention
KI15 **Zhong Zhu 中注** **Central Flow**	Reunion point with Chong Mai	Physical, mental and sexual fatigue
KI16 **Huang Shu肓俞** **Abdominal Point**	Disposal of the turbid Ye Fluids by the Large Intestine; Reunion point with Chong Mai	Constipation or diarrhea; anal fissures; problems during childbirth; Phlegm in the upper burner
KI2 **Ran Gu 然谷** **Blazing Valley**	Activation of the relationship between Kidney and the Bao; Departure point for Yin Qiao Mai	Low back pain and knee pain; diarrhea, cystitis; sleep apnea in obese patients
CV2 Qu Gu 曲骨 **Curved Bone or CV6** **Qi Hai 氣海 Sea of Qi** **with moxa**	Disposal of the impure Fluids by the Lower Burner (Large Intestine and Urinary Bladder)	Dampness in the Lower Burner

(Contd.....

Acupoint	Action	Symptoms
LR13 Zhang Men 章門 **Door of Shelter** **GB26 Dai Mai** 帶脈 **Belt Vessel** **GB27 Wu Shu** 五樞 **Fifth Pivot** **GB28 Wei Dao** 維道 **Meeting Path**	Disposal of Dampness by Dai Mai	Dampness in the Lower Burner
GB41 + **GB26 +** **KI16**	Consolidation and tonification of Jing by Dai Mai	Male infertility with hemorrhoids, anal fissures and fistulas, pilonidal cysts, *etc.*
BL43 + **KI16 +** **BL53 +** **GB41**	Consolidation of Gao and descent of Jing to the Bao	Male infertility with asthenozoospermia
LI16 + **ST36 +** **KI11**	Descent of turbid Ye Fluids from the Lungo to the Bao	Male infertility with oligozoospermia
LI14 with moxa + **ST36 +** **KI13**	Descent of Lung Blood to the Bao	Infertility
BL31 + **BL32 +** **BL33 +** **BL34**	Nourishment of Jing-Seed and Jing-Marrow *via* the Blood	Infertility

Legend: LUTS: Lower Urinary Tract Symptoms; The names of the points are from ChineseMedicineWiki.org

APPENDIX 4

AZOOSPERMIA

Kidney Yang deficiency:modified ***Bu tian yu ling dan***
Kidney Yin deficiency with Empty Heat:modified ***Shen sui yu lin dan***
Blood stasis blocks the Channel: modified ***Xie fu zhu yu tang***
Damp-Heat, Phlegm and Stasis block the Channel: modified ***Wu shen tang***and ***Xiao luo wan***

ASTHENOZOOSPERMIA

Kidney Qi deficiency: modified ***Huang jing zan yu dan*** and ***Wu zi yan zong wan***
Kidney Jing deficiency: modified ***Qi bao mei ran dan***
Spleen and Stomach deficiency: modified ***Bu zhong yi qi tang***
Damp-Heat block the Lower Burner: modified ***Bi xie fen qing yin***
Obstruction of the Collaterals: modified ***Tao hong si wu tang***

AUTOIMMUNE INFERTILITY

Yin deficiency with Yin Fire:modified ***Dang gui liu huang tang***
Obstruction of the Collaterals and the sperm cannot get out: modified ***Tuo li xiao du san***
Spleen and Qi Wei deficiency:modified ***Yu ping san***and ***Shen ling bai zhu san***
Damp-Heat:modified ***Wu shen tang***

OLIGOZOOSPERMIA

Kidney Jing deficiency:modified ***Ju jing tang***
Kidney Yang deficiency:modified ***Wu zi yan zong*** and modified ***You gui wan***
Spleen Qi deficiency: modified ***Bu zhong yi qi tang***
Damp-Heat in the Lower Burner: modified***Bei xie fen qing yin***
Qi stagnation and Blood stasis:modified ***Xue fu zhu yu tang***

ABNORMALITIES IN SEMEN LIQUEFACTION

Kidney Yin deficiency:modified ***Zhi bai di huang wan***
Kidney Yang deficiency:modified ***Ba ji er xian tang***
Damp-Heat:modified ***Bei xie fen qing yin***

APPENDIX 5

REFERENCE VALUES OF LABORATORY DIAGNOSTIC TESTS IN MALE INFERTILITY

Hormones	Conventional values	SI Units	Increase	Decrease
DHT	30–86 ng/dL	1.0–2.9 nmol/L	Exercise, hemoconcentration	Immobilisation, postprandial
Estradiol	10–60 ng/L	25–220 pmol/L	Smoking, hemoconcentration, after age 55	Malnutrition, frequent intense physical exercise
FSH	5–15 mIU/mL	5–25 IU/L	Ketoconazole, L-dopa, clomiphene	Obesity, malnutrition, phenotiazine
LH	0–18 mIU/L	0–18.0 UI/L	Kidney failure; propranolol, ketoconazole, clomiphene	Obesity, fasting, acute disease, intense exercise; propranolol, exogenous testosterone
Inhibin B	Adults: 50–250 pg/mL			
17OH progesterone	< 4.0 ug/L	1.2–12 nmol/L	Ketoconazole, ACTH	
Prolactin	2–15 ug/L	84–520 pmol/L	Stress, physical exercise, smoking, postprandial, renal failure	Aging; L-dopa, ergot alkaloids
Total testosterone	300–1000 ng/dL	10.4–34.7 nmol/L	Hemoconcentration, physical exercise, postprandial; barbiturates, clomiphene	Stress, frequent intense physical exercise; exogenous androgens, spironolactone, tetrahydrocannabinol, ketoconazole
Free testosterone	7.5–41.0 ng/dL	0.18–1.42 nmol/L	Same as testosterone	Same as testosterone
SHBG	0.2–1.4 ug/dL	10–70 nmol/L	Hemoconcentration; thyroid hormones, antiepileptic drugs	Obesity; exogenous androgens

Legend: DHT = Dihydrotestosterone; FSH = follicle stimulating hormone; LH = luteinizing hormone; SHBG = sex hormone binding globulin.

Note: the reference values can change depending on the system employed for the measurement; it is thus necessary to check the reference values of the laboratory which performed the assay.

(Contd.....

Spermiogram:	5th percentile	50th percentile
Volume (mL)	1.5	3.7
Number of sperm (10^6/ejaculate)	39	255
Concentration of sperm (10^6/mL)	15	73
Progressive motility (PR, %)	32	55
Non-progressive motility (NP, %)	1	5
Total motility (PR+NP, %)	40	61
Immobile sperm (IM, %)	22	39
Vitality (%)	58	79
Normal forms (%)	4	15

The spermiogram reference values are distributed according to the percentages of men whose partners became pregnant within 12 months after discontinuation of oral contraceptives; 5th percentile = 5% of fertile men had those values; 50th percentile = 50% of fertile men had those values.

APPENDIX 6

ALBUGINEA   Envelope of fibrous connective tissue of the testis.

AMH   (AntiMullerian Hormone) Hormone produced by Sertoli cells. It promotes apoptosis of mullerian structures and genital differentiation into a male phenotype.

ANDROGEN BINDING PROTEIN   (ABP) Glycoprotein produced by Sertoli cells that transports testosterone dihydrotestosterone and 17-beta estradiol.

ANEJACULATION   Inability to ejaculate.

ANEUPLOIDY   Altered number of chromosomes present in a cell.

ASPERMIA   Absence of ejaculate.

ASTHENOZOOSPERMIA   Percentage of sperm with progressive motility (PR) below the lower limit.

AZOOSPERMIA   Absence of sperm in the ejaculate.

CAG REPEATS   Polymorphic region of CAG triplets repeat on the gene of the androgen receptor.

CAIS   (Complete Androgen Insensitivity). Also known as Morris syndrome it is a form of complete insensitivity to androgens due to a mutation of the androgen receptor, with female external genitalia at birth.

CFTR   (Cystic fibrosis transmembrane conductance regulator). Gene whose mutations cause cystic fibrosis.

CORPUS CAVERNOSUS   One of the two elongated masses of erectile tissue that are located on each side and on the back of the penis. They are surrounded by the tunica albuginea.

CRYOPRESERVATION   Procedure used to store embryos or gametes at very low temperature (in liquid nitrogen).

CRYPTOZOOSPERMIA   Sperm is absent in the fresh ejaculate but is present in the pellet after centrifugation.

CRYPTORCHIDISM   The testicle is outside of the scrotum because of an anomaly of its descent.

CYTOGENETICS   Branch of genetics and cytology which deals with the study of chromosomes.

DIHYDROTESTOSTERONE   (DHT). Androgen hormone synthesised from testosterone by the enzyme Type 2 5-alpha-reductase. It has a bigger affinity for the androgenic receptor than testosterone.

DIPLOID   Chromosomal structure characterized by the presence of two couples for each chromosome (46 chromosomes).

EJACULATE   The combination of seminal fluid sperm, and of the other cells present in the seminal fluid.

EPIDIDYMIS   Cord-like structure arranged on the posterior and superior edge of the testis (didymus). It contains a convoluted channel about 4–6 meters long where the spermatozoa undergo the final maturation.

FSH (Follicle Stimulating Hormone). Gonadotropin produced by the pituitary which stimulates Sertoli cells and spermatogenesis.

GAMETE Mature cell that participates in sexual reproduction.

GIFT (Gamete Intra-Fallopian-Transfer). Transfer of gametes inside the Fallopian tubes.

GONADOTROPINS Hormones secreted by the hypophysis under hypothalamic control for the regulation of the reproductive function (FSH and LH).

HAPLOID Chromosomal arrangement characterized by the presence of a single set of chromosomes (23 chromosomes).

HEMATOSPERMIA Presence of red blood cells in the ejaculate.

HYDROCELE Acute or chronic swelling of the scrotum and/or groin due to the accumulation of fluid in the tunica vaginalis of the testis.

HYPOGONADISM Condition of inadequate gonadal function which is manifested by an insufficient gametogenesis and/or secretion of androgenic hormones.

HYPOPHYSIS Endocrine gland in the lower part of the brain consisting of two areas (neurohypophysis and adenohypophysis). The adenohypophysis produces gonadotropins.

HYPOTHALAMUS Brain area which controls and regulates many other brain areas including adenohypophysis.

ICSI (Intra-Cytoplasmic Sperm Injection). Sperm injection inside the cytoplasm of the egg cell.

INFERTILITY Inability of a couple to achieve pregnancy after one year of constant and unprotected sexual intercourse; it is primary when the person or the couple have never been able to conceive and secondary when the infertile subject or couple have already conceived in the past.

INHIBIN Hormone produced by the Sertoli cells that inhibits the production of FSH at the pituitary level; it is considered a marker of spermatogenesis.

LEUKOCYTOSPERMIA Presence of leukocytes in the ejaculate above the reference value.

LEYDIG CELLS Cells localized in the tubular interstitium specialized in the secretion of testosterone.

LH (Luteinizing Hormone). Gonadotropin produced by the pituitary which regulates the secretion of testosterone by the testicular Leydig cells (steroidogenesis).

LHRH (LH releasing hormone). Hypothalamic hormone which induces the release of LH from the anterior hypophysis.

LUTS (Lower Urinary Tract Symptoms). Group of symptoms which indicate a dysfunction of the lower urinary tract.

MAIS (Mild Androgen Insensitivity). Mild form of androgen insensitivity due to a mutation of the androgenic receptor with male external genitalia at birth.

MEIOSIS Process of cell division leading to the formation of cells with a halved chromosomal set (haploid).

MESA Microsurgical Epidydimal Sperm Aspiration.

MTHFR (Methylene tetrahydrofolate reductase). Rate-limiting enzyme in the methyl cycle which transforms homocysteine into methionine.

MUTATION The variant allele is present in <1% of the general population.

NECROZOOSPERMIA Low percentage of live sperm and/or high percentage of immobile sperm in the ejaculate.

OLIGOZOOSPERMIA Total number or concentration of sperm in the ejaculate below the threshold values.

ORCHITIS Inflammation of the testes.

PAIS (Partial Androgen Insensitivity) or Reifenstein syndrome, is a partial form of androgen insensitivity due to a mutation of the androgenic receptor, with ambiguous external genitalia at birth.

POLYMORPHISM The variant allele is present in >1% of the general population.

PREMATURE EJACULATION Ejaculation is premature when it occurs before the person wishes due to a strong and persistent absence of reasonable voluntary control of ejaculation and orgasm during sexual activity.

PYOSPERMIA Abnormally high concentration of white blood cells in the ejaculate as caused by a bacterial infection.

RETROGRADE EJACULATION Abnormal ejaculation with a backward flow of semen into the bladder.

SEMEN (Or sperm) The organic substance emitted during ejaculation consisting of seminal plasma and spermatozoa.

SEMINAL FLUID (Or seed or sperm). The organic liquid substance emitted through ejaculation composed of the sperm and seminal plasma.

SERTOLI CELLS Cells localized in the wall of the seminiferous tubules with the function of supporting spermatogenesis.

SF-1 (Steroidogenic Factor 1). Gene responsible for the beginning of the male differentiation of the gonad.

SOX-9 (SRY-related HMG box). Gene responsible for the beginning of the male differentiation of the gonad.

SPERM (Or semen). The organic substance emitted during ejaculation consisting of seminal plasma and spermatozoa.

SPERMATOGENESIS The process of sperm formation starting from the differentiation of the male germ cells.

SPERMIATION The process of sperm release from the lumen of the seminiferous tubules at the end of spermatogenesis.

SRY (Sex Determining Region Y). Gene responsible for the beginning of the male differentiation of the gonad.

STERILITY One or both members of a couple have a permanent physical condition which makes conception impossible.

STEROIDOGENESIS Synthesis of steroid hormones.

STW (Seminal Tract Washout). Surgical techniques which retrieves sperm by washing the vas deferens.

TERATOZOOSPERMIA Percentage of morphologically normal sperm below the reference values.

TESA TEsticular Sperm Aspiration.

TESE TEsticular Sperm Extraction.

TESTOSTERONE Main androgenic hormone responsible for the development of the male genital system and male sexual characteristics.

TET Tubal Embryo Transfer.

TRUE HERMAPHRODITISM Male and female gonads are present at the same time in the same organism.

VAS DEFERENS Continuation of the epididymal ducts of the testis; they end at the base of the prostate as ejaculatory ducts.

ZIFT Zygote Intrafallopian Transfer.

ZYGOTE Fertilized oocyte which has not yet undergone segmentation.

APPENDIX 7

ACRONYMS USED IN THE TEXT

ABP　Androgen Binding Protein

ACTH　Adreno CorticoTropic Hormone

AFP　Alfa Feto Protein

AMH　Anti Mullerian Hormone

AZF　AZoospermia Factor

AR　Androgen Receptor

ALT　ALanina amino Transferase

ART　Assisted Reproductive Technology

ASA　Anti Sperm Antibodies

AST　ASpartato Transaminase

BMI　Body Mass Index

CAG　trinucleotide repeat Cytosine-Adenine-Guanine

CAIS　Complete Androgen Insensitivity Syndrome

CB1 and CB2　endocannabinoid receptors

CEA　CarcinoEmbryonic Antigen

CFTR　Cystic Fibrosis Transmembrane Conductance Regulator

CHD7　Chromodomain Helicase DNA binding protein 7

COPD　Chronic Obstructive Pulmonary Disease

DDE　Dichloro-Diphenyl dichloro-Ethylene

DDT　Dichloro-Diphenyl Trichloroethane

DHT　DiHydroTestosterone

DNA　DeoxyriboNucleic Acid

FGF　Fibroblast Growth Factor

FGFR1　Fibroblast Growth Factor Receptor 1

FISH　Fluorescence In Situ Hybridization

FSH　Follicle Stimulating Hormone

FT4　Free Thyroxine

GDNF　Glial-Derived Neurotrophic Factor

GH　Growth Hormone

GIFT　Gamete Intra-Fallopian Transfer

GnRH　Gonadotropin Release Hormone

GnRHR　Gonadotropin Release Hormone Receptor

GPR54 G Protein-coupled Receptor 54

hCG human Chorionic Gonadotropin

HIV Human Immunodeficiency Virus

HPV Human Papilloma Virus

HSV Herpes Simplex Virus

ICI Intra Cervical Insemination

ICSI Intra Cytoplasmic Sperm Injection

IFN Interferon

IGF Insulin Growth Factor

IHH Idiopatic Hypogonadic Hypogonadism

IPI Intra Peritoneal Insemination

IUI Intra Uterine Insemination

IVF *In Vitro* Fertilization

KiSS1 KiSSpeptin gene

KL Kit Ligand

LDH Lactate DeHydrogenase

LH Luteinizing Hormone

LHRH Luteinizing Hormone-Releasing Hormone

LIH Leucemia Inhibitory Factor

LUTS Lower Urinary Tract Symptoms

MAIS Mild Androgen Insensitivity Syndrome

MAR test Mixed Antiglobulin Reaction test

MESA Microsurgical Epididimal Sperm Aspiration

MSVA MicroSurgical Vas Aspiration

MSY Male Specific Y

MTHFR Metilene Tetra Hydro Folate Reductase

NP Non Progressive sperm motility

NSAIDs NonSteroidal Anti-Inflammatory Drugs

NSE Neuron Specific Enolase

OAT Oligo-Astheno-Teratozoospermia

PAIS Partial Androgen Insensitivity Syndrome

PDGF Platelet-Derived Growth Factor

PESA Percutaneous Epididimal Sperm Aspiration

PLAP Placental Alkaline Phosphatase

PR	PRogressive sperm motility
PROK2	PROKineticin 2
PROKR2	PROKineticin 2 Receptor
PVC	PolyVinyl Chloride
SCF	Stem Cell Factor
SF-1	Steroidogenic Factor 1
SHBG	Sex Hormone Binding Globulin
SNiPs	Single Nucleotide Polymorphisms
SOX-9	SRY-related HMG box
SRY	Sex Determining Region Y
STD	Sexually Transmitted Diseases
STW	Seminal Tract Washout
TAC3	TAChykinin 3
TACR3	TAChykinin 3 Receptor
TESA	TEsticular Sperm Aspiration
TESE	TEsticular Sperm Extraction
TET	Tubal Embryo Transfer
TGF	Transforming Growth Factor
TNF	Tumor Necrosis Factor
TRUSCA	TRansrectal Ultrasonically-guided Sperm Cyst Aspiration
TSH	Thyroid Stimulating Hormone
TUNEL	(Terminal deoxynucleotidyl transferase dUTP Nick End Labeling)
VNTR	Variable Number of Tandem Repeats
ZIFT	Zigote Intrafallopian Transfer

SUBJECT INDEX